Praise for Charlie Morley

'Charlie Morley, a lucid dreaming expert, offers simple techniques to help you master the skill.'
The Guardian

'Learning from Charlie felt like him taking me by the hand and guiding me on an exploration of my own mind. I highly recommend him not only for his knowledge of the subject matter but more so for his unique ability to teach in a fun and compelling way that gets results for his students.'
Vishen Lakhiani, New York Times bestselling author and founder of Mindvalley

'Joyfully exploring consciousness, lucid dreaming and Buddhism, Charlie Morley gently stretches the reader's mind to accept dream yoga's premise of real awakening. I recommend this for everyone on the lucid dreaming path.'
Robert Waggoner, author of Lucid Dreaming: Gateway to the Inner Self

'This is pioneering work: a lucid dreaming guide that masterfully bridges the gap between science and practical application, offering an impactful exploration into the potential of lucid dreams. It is an indispensable tool for anyone aspiring to explore and transform their conscious experience through the art of lucid dreaming. I will recommend to my patients.'
Dr Heather Sequeira, consultant chartered psychologist

'Partnering with Charlie in our research has truly been a rewarding journey. I hold him in high esteem, and I'm delighted to find his unique blend of wisdom, wit and wonder shining through in this book.'
Dr Garret Yount, molecular neurobiologist, Institute of Noetic Science

'Wow! Charlie Morley has concocted a powerful mix of spirituality and scientific research to reveal how the mystery of sleep can wake you up to a whole new life.'
Robert Holden, PhD, author of Shift Happens!

T0188600

'Charlie's pioneering work on mindfulness of sleep and dream has already delivered great results within the UK Defence community. I am hugely grateful to Charlie for the work he has already done and I know will continue to do.'
Lt General R.A. Magowan CB, CBE, Deputy Commander UK Strategic Command and Commandant General Royal Marines

'In Dreams of Awakening Charlie shares wonderful advice, not just for dreaming but also for living – and he has a knack for conveying a modern take on ancient wisdom clearly and compellingly.'
Professor Ken Paller, cognitive neuroscientist, Northwestern University, Illinois

'Charlie Morley has the beautiful ability to present authentic practices in accessible ways. His dedication, knowledge and kindness shine throughout and I firmly believe this book will bring great benefit to those who read it. He is an inspiration to those who wish to understand spirituality.'
Eddy Elsey, bestselling author of Let Healing Happen

'I have run joint retreats with Charlie and I consider him to be the most experienced and authentic practitioner of lucid dreaming teaching in Europe. He has been training since his teens and this book offers a training programme based on this unique practical experience.'
Rob Nairn, author of Living, Dreaming, Dying

'Charlie is proof of evolution. He's the next generation – sharp of mind and sweet of heart. He's like a DJ mixing old and new to create a practice that's relevant, useful and most importantly, one that works. I wholeheartedly recommend his book. He's the real thing.'
Ya'Acov Darling Khan, co-author of Movement Medicine: How to Awaken, Dance and Live Your Dreams

DREAMS
OF
AWAKENING

Also by Charlie Morley

Books

Do the Shadow Work (2024)
Wake Up to Sleep (2021)
Lucid Dreaming Made Easy (2018)
Dreaming Through Darkness (2017)

Guided Meditations
Available on the *Empower You Unlimited Audio* app

Lucid Dreaming, Conscious Sleeping
7 Days to Great Sleep

Online Courses

Lucid Dreaming Made Easy

DREAMS OF AWAKENING

Use Lucid Dreaming to Rewire Your Brain While You Sleep

CHARLIE MORLEY

HAY HOUSE

Carlsbad, California • New York City
London • Sydney • New Delhi

Published in the United Kingdom by:
Hay House UK Ltd, The Sixth Floor, Watson House
54 Baker Street, London W1U 7BU
Tel: +44 (0)20 3927 7290; www.hayhouse.co.uk

Published in the United States of America by:
Hay House LLC, PO Box 5100, Carlsbad, CA 92018-5100
Tel: (1) 760 431 7695 or (800) 654 5126; www.hayhouse.com

Published in Australia by:
Hay House Australia Publishing Pty Ltd, 18/36 Ralph St, Alexandria NSW 2015
Tel: (61) 2 9669 4299; www.hayhouse.com.au

Published in India by:
Hay House Publishers (India) Pvt Ltd, Muskaan Complex, Plot No.3, B-2,
Vasant Kunj, New Delhi 110 070
Tel: (91) 11 4176 1620; www.hayhouse.co.in

A catalogue record for this book is available from the British Library.

Tradepaper ISBN: 978-1-4019-7814-3
E-book ISBN: 978-1-83782-238-6
Audiobook ISBN: 978-1-83782-239-3

Interior illustrations: 1, 65, 177: Glitch Lab App/Unsplash; 23: Keith Hearne; 59: Paul Wootton; 76: Charlie Morley; 202: Dr Garret Yount

10 9 8 7 6 5 4 3 2 1

Printed in the United States of America

This product uses responsibly sourced papers and/or recycled materials. For more information, see www.hayhouse.com.

*For the dakinis, the awakened women
to whom I owe so much.*

And especially for my Muma, 1954–2023.

CONTENTS

Foreword by Lama Yeshe Rinpoche   xi

Introduction   xiii

PART I: GROUND

Chapter 1:   The Basics   3

Chapter 2:   The Science of Lucidity   21

Chapter 3:   The Psychological Benefits of Lucid Dreaming   29

Chapter 4:   Sleeping Buddhas   45

Chapter 5:   The Spiritual Benefits of Lucid Dreaming   55

PART II: PATH

Chapter 6:   Daytime Lucid Dreaming Techniques   67

Chapter 7:   Lucidity in Action: Top 10 Dream Plans   99

Chapter 8:   Night-time Lucid Dreaming Techniques   127

Chapter 9:   Liminal State Techniques   157

PART III: GERMINATION

Chapter 10: Embracing the Obstacles of the Night   179

Chapter 11: Treating PTSD Lucidly   193

Chapter 12: Blurring the Boundaries   205

Chapter 13: Beyond Lucidity   225

Chapter 14: Awakening within the Dream   243

Appendix I: Mindfulness Meditation   249

Appendix II: A Selection of Lucid Dreams and Clarity Dreams   257

References   287

Bibliography   299

Acknowledgements   303

Index   305

About the Author   317

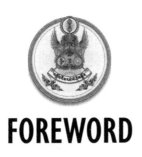

FOREWORD

Buddhist meditation is ultimately about liberating the mind from illusion and self-deception. To this end, it is necessary to train the mind and develop kindness, compassion and wisdom. The dreaming mind is fertile ground for developing these qualities. In the Tibetan tradition, the refined discipline of dream yoga has been practised for 1,000 years, and as one of the famous Six Yogas of Naropa, it is an important element in our intensive four-year retreats at Samye Ling monastery. The stability of the lucid dream is the foundation of dream yoga.

In *Dreams of Awakening*, Charlie Morley is offering a useful, practical synthesis of both Western and Tibetan Buddhist approaches to dream work, and the Western methods of inducing lucid dreams are a significant support for anyone wishing to engage in the practice of dream yoga in the future.

I am one of Charlie's teachers and have a strong connection with him; through this, I have confidence in his honest simplicity and trust his methods. His clarity, humility and humanity make it easier for people to understand his presentation of the deep and important subject of lucid dreaming, and I am satisfied that people who study this book and attend his courses can trust him. Charlie's approach is particularly valuable because he is offering methods of working with dreaming that will help people in societies where relevant methods have until now been lacking.

It's now over 10 years since *Dreams of Awakening* was first published and I hope this new edition will continue to help people with an interest in learning more about lucid dreaming and the benefits this can bring to their lives.

I recommend this book to anyone who wishes to benefit from living a more awakened life.

Lama Yeshe Losal Rinpoche
Chairman of the Rokpa Trust
Abbot of Kagyu Samye Ling
Executive Director of the Holy Isle Project

INTRODUCTION

In 1881, the American astronomer E.E. Barnard discovered a new galaxy. At the time, it wasn't recognized as a galaxy, because the notion of multiple galaxies was deemed ridiculous. There was only one galaxy – ours. The Milky Way was the entire universe. A couple of decades into the 20th century, it was finally conceded that there could be up to a dozen galaxies, although many people still thought this impossible. We now know that there are over 100 billion galaxies just in the tiny section of the universe that we know about. From one galaxy to 100 billion galaxies in one lifetime. And we dare to think that something doesn't exist simply because we haven't seen it yet?

Lord Kelvin, the Nobel laureate 15 years before Einstein, told his university students not to study post-graduate physics because there was nothing left to discover. He thought they had nailed it already. And then a decade or so later came relativity and quantum mechanics. Oops.

We humans have got form when it comes to dismissing that which we are yet to discover. And so it was with lucid dreaming until relatively recently. But now lucid dreaming is not only accepted as a scientifically verifiable phenomenon, it has actually been described by Professor Matthew Walker in his book *Why We Sleep* as the next step in human evolution. In fact, Walker joked in a podcast recently, 'We don't need to be worried about AI, we need to be worried about lucid dreamers becoming the next super-race of humanity!'[1]

The world has changed so much since 2013, when I wrote the first edition of this book: smartphones are in every pocket, gender is no longer seen as binary, Instagram, Tinder and TikTok happened, world peace didn't, AI is here to stay and so are UFOs. Oh, and I turned 40.

So, it was with the eyes of early middle age that I read back over what I wrote in my late twenties and, with the discernment that the newly grey hairs on my head have given me, cut entire sections and added whole new chapters. We needed to keep the wordcount pretty much the same as the first edition, so I removed a lot of the less important parts to make way for the new stuff. You'll be able to find most of the cut sections in PDF format on my website, though.

The book has been fully revised, restructured and rewritten, and although it keeps the same title, it really is quite different from the original. Some of the techniques that were barely mentioned in the first edition take centre stage now, due to 15 years of teaching experience proving their effectiveness. The new sections on PTSD treatment, inner child work and using lucid dreaming for depression and grief were missing from the first edition simply because I wasn't aware that they were possible 10 years ago.

Using the same three-part structure of Ground, Path and Germination, my aim is to offer a map based on almost 25 years of lucid dreaming experience that, if followed, will allow the recognition of the dream state to become the recognition of your mind's true potential.

After a solid grounding in the history, context and benefits of lucid dreaming within both Western and Buddhist traditions, we'll set off down the path of learning how to be mindfully aware in our dreams and sleep. Then finally we'll explore the germination of the practice, journey into the frontier lands and see just how deep the rabbit-hole goes.

The journey won't be just in reading this book, but in where it will inspire you to go. So, let's set off on the road… to dreams of awakening.

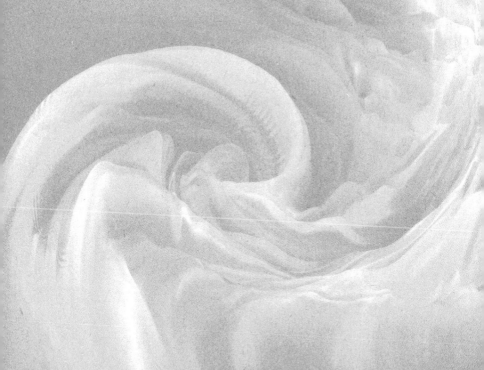

PART I

GROUND

CHAPTER 1

THE BASICS

'Let us learn to dream, and then we
may perhaps find the truth.'

Friedrich Kekulé

Lucid dreaming is magical and misunderstood in equal measure. That's why it's useful to have a stable ground of understanding before applying the practice. So, let's prepare our ground, weed out the facts from the fiction and open our minds to the limitless potential of the field before us.

What Is a Lucid Dream?

To start by clarifying terms, a lucid dream is a dream in which we are actively aware that we are dreaming as the dream is happening. From a psychological point of view, a lucid dream could be described as 'the reactivation of self-reflective awareness within the previously non-aware REM dreaming sleep state'.

But don't be deceived by this dry definition. Lucid dreams are commonly described as among the most thrilling experiences to be had. A fully lucid dream isn't a hazy, imprecise phantasmagoria, but a full-colour, high-definition and hyper-realistic experience. It can profoundly reconfigure our perception of reality.

Once we become lucid, we don't wake up – we're still sound asleep – but parts of our brain become reactivated (the right dorsolateral prefrontal cortex primarily),[1] allowing us to experience the dream state consciously and choose what we want to do in it. We can now direct the dream at will.

Once lucid, we're not half-awake/half-asleep, we're not just having a very vivid dream and we're not having an out-of-body experience (sometimes called astral projection). We're simply conscious and aware while in REM dreaming sleep.

About 55 per cent of people report having had a lucid dream at least once in their lives and only 23 per cent report having them monthly,[2] but lucid dreaming is a learnable skill and my job is to teach you how.

From a Buddhist perspective, lucid dreaming is seen as a form of mind training in which we learn to consciously recognize our dreams as a way to train our mind to be more awake and aware and kinder in everyday life. To dream lucidly is to live lucidly – to wake up to life.

The term 'lucid dream' was supposedly coined by Frederik van Eeden, a Dutch psychiatrist, over 100 years ago,[3] but is misleading. My workshop participants sometimes describe a particularly intense, vivid dream they have had and ask whether this could be classified as a lucid dream. My answer is always that if you have to ask whether a dream was lucid, it probably wasn't. When you've had a fully lucid dream, you won't be left wondering if it qualified.

To avoid this confusion, some have put forward the alternative term 'conscious dreaming'. But the word 'lucid' originally conveyed the meaning of 'having insight', rather than describing the perceptual quality of the experience. It is this element of insight that is the cornerstone of the lucid dream. In fact, it reveals the profound potential of the mind in a way that few other states of consciousness can, because through lucid dreaming we become aware of awareness itself.

As mentioned previously, this awakening of awareness within the dream state isn't accompanied by any physiological awakening. To all outward appearances, we're still sound asleep and 'unconscious', yet internally, in our dreaming mind, it could be said that we are wide awake. Van Eeden commented, 'In lucid dreams the sleeper remembers his daily life [and] reaches a state of perfect awareness... Yet the sleep is undisturbed, deep and refreshing.'[4]

It seems a contradiction to be both aware and asleep at the same time, and this neurological paradox means that it was only in the late 1970s that lucid dreaming came to be verified by Western scientific means.

Although Western science was quite late to the game, the first academic article on lucid dreaming was published in 1948 in an edition of *Psychiatric Quarterly*[5] under the title 'Pleasant Dreams!', and lucid dreaming has been a scientifically verified phenomenon for almost 50 years now. It has unique and 'discernible neural correlates', which means that it's not just psychological, it's physical, and yet there are still some people who question its validity, so let's go a little deeper into some of the scientific proof of lucid dreaming.

Studies from Frankfurt University's neurological clinic and the Max Planck Institute of Psychiatry have found that specific alterations to brain physiology appear once a dreamer becomes lucid. Using brain-imaging technology such as magnetic resonance tomography and EEG, scientists can now pinpoint the actual 'Aha! I'm dreaming!' moment of lucid awareness and its neurophysiological correlates. The researchers concluded that: 'Lucid dreaming constitutes a hybrid state of consciousness with definable and measurable differences from the waking state and from the REM [rapid eye movement] dream state.'[6] They discovered that when lucid consciousness was attained within the dream, activity in areas associated with self-assessment and self-perception increased markedly within seconds.[7]

How did this actually work? When the subject was asleep and dreaming non-lucidly, the researchers observed that their prefrontal cortex (an area linked to our sense of self and agency) was almost entirely offline, but when they became lucid, that area became reactivated, as their sense of self switched back on and they went, 'Aha! I'm dreaming!' This means the apparent paradox of being both aware and asleep, which had previously caused a lot of resistance and scepticism in the scientific establishment, was simply a failure to understand how two distinct brain regions could be activated simultaneously.

The Brain Thinks We're Awake

Here is an interesting philosophical question: is conscious awareness predicated on being physically awake? No, not for the brain. From a neurological point of view, self-reflective consciousness is predicated on prefrontal cortex activation, regardless of what state of waking or sleep we're in.

This means that, to our psycho-physical system, a lucid dream isn't just a visualization, it's a reality, and because of this, neural pathways can be created and strengthened in our lucid dreams, just as they can while we're awake. This is due to neuroplasticity: The more we use certain brain networks, the more blood flow they receive and the deeper the grooves in the grey-matter density of that brain region become. This means that – audacious as it may sound – through lucid dreaming we can actually rewire our brain, and so create new habits of mind, get better at waking-state activities and make lasting changes to our neurology while we sleep.

The implications of this are huge. If our neurological system doesn't differentiate between waking and lucid dreaming experiences, if we integrate a trauma in a lucid dream or have a spiritual breakthrough, does our brain think that we have actually done so in real life? Yes, and that is the core neurological process underlying the huge transformational potential of lucid dreaming.

Charlie says

'Interestingly, because of this, the idea of "Pinch yourself to see if you're dreaming" doesn't work in a lucid dream and instead most people simply feel the pain of the pinch. This is nuts, because nothing is actually being pinched (it's just your dream fingers pinching your dream arm), and yet your brain still creates the illusion of pain. Buddha was right: "With our mind we make the world!"'

Realer than Real

The thing that surprises most first-time lucid dreamers is the fact that fully lucid dreams aren't very dreamy at all. The lucid dream state both looks and feels real. It is a meticulously intricate mental construct that often appears as realistic as our waking reality. It may, in fact, seem so real that we come to question our perceptions of waking reality and stand in awe of the creative aptitude of the human mind. Since I started training, I've had hundreds of lucid dreams and yet I'm still struck by the infinite potential of lucid dreaming and its capacity to facilitate entire dimensions of 'reality' within our own mind. The lucid dream environment is often so meticulously realistic that some new lucid dreamers come to the audacious conclusion that it can't be a dream at all and they must have travelled to another dimension. And indeed they have – a dimension within their own mind.

Does this mean lucid dreamers stand to lose touch with reality? No, in fact quite the opposite: once we can penetrate the persuasive reality of the dreamscape and know it as an illusion, we become better equipped to recognize self-deception in the waking state. This makes us more grounded and more aware.

If you haven't had a lucid dream yet, or are still unsure as to what one actually constitutes, take a moment now to check out some of the lucid dreams at the back of the book. Please do take a moment to do this.*

Essentially, during a lucid dream the mind is creating an incredibly detailed three-dimensional projection to form the functional reality of the dreamscape, while another part of the mind is consciously interacting with this projection in real time. So, in a lucid dream we are both the creator and the created, the projector and the projected.

This mind-boggling process reveals the infinite potential of the brain in a way few other states of consciousness can, because through lucid dreaming we become conscious within our unconscious. This opens up the possibility of directly interacting with psychological aspects and archetypes at a seemingly tangible level.

This allows us to literally dialogue with the source of our deepest fear or have a discussion with the personification of our own mind.

Charlie says

'I will never forget the first time I intentionally did this. It changed my life forever. It was the dream in which I met the personification of my subconscious mind. She hugged me and gave me a kind of pep talk!' (For a full description of this dream, see Dream 8, page 266.)

Being conscious in the unconscious mind means that we are in a state not dissimilar to hypnotherapeutic trance, and in fact anything that can be treated by hypnotherapy can also be treated by lucid dreaming: addictions, phobias, depression, sports performance,

---

* Not everybody likes to read through other people's lucid dreams (which is why I haven't included any in the main body of the text), but I have provided a selection of my own for those that do.

confidence issues, physical ailments and even post-traumatic stress disorder.

And, just as a hypnotherapist might plant a beneficial suggestion of healing intent into our unconscious mind, a lucid dreamer might do the same, but due to the even deeper depths to which lucid dreaming takes us, it can work even more powerfully.

My friend the lucid dreaming expert Robert Waggoner once told me, 'Lucid dreaming helps us to see the magic that already exists.' It's true: while we are learning to see through illusion, lucid dreaming nonetheless gives us a tangible experience of the magic of the dream state. We find ourselves experiencing a huge three-dimensional virtual-reality simulation of our own psyche, in which we aren't just one with everything, we *are* everything. We are the main player in a hallucinatory projection of our own mind in which psychological concepts such as love, fear and time can be met and dialogued with in personified form.

In a fully lucid dream, the quality of cognitive awareness allows us to interact directly with the dream and to influence it. Given enough lucidity, we can experience a dream with exactly the same reflective awareness as when we are awake. We know that we are actually asleep in our bed, we remember what we had planned to do once lucid and we know that we are moving around our own psyche.

Lucid dreams are shown to differ from ordinary (REM) dreams by an increased brain frequency in the 40Hz (or gamma) range in the frontal and frontolateral areas of the brain. Gamma brainwaves are the highest-frequency brainwaves and are associated with high levels of insight and awareness, peak concentration and spiritual experience. This increase in gamma activity allows us to access a level of awareness not just equal to the waking state, but actually much higher.

Lucid dreaming isn't an easy skill to learn, but it is undeniably one of the most exciting and rewarding practices we may ever engage in, with a wealth of both psychological and spiritual benefits. Within the safety of our *bodhicitta* motivation (more about that later), it's a completely safe practice, open to all ages and abilities, offering a unique insight into our own psychology.

In a letter to a mourning friend, Albert Einstein wrote, 'A human being... experiences himself, his thoughts and feelings as something separated from the rest – a kind of optical delusion of his consciousness... To try to overcome this delusion is the way to attain true peace of mind.'[8]

Through lucid dreaming we can overcome this delusion, as we experience a fully realistic 'reality' that may seem separate from us, but which we know we are dreaming into existence and is actually within us. Thus we are introduced, in visceral fashion, to the radical notion that duality may be a delusion. In a lucid dream we are one with everything, because we *are* everything. This experience can help dissolve our sense of isolation in the waking state, allowing us to finally wake up to the Oneness on which Einstein and the mystics of the ages have been so eloquent.

What Is the Lucidity Spectrum?

Although full lucidity depends upon an 'Aha!' moment in which we realize we're dreaming, followed by the ability to direct the dream at will, there is a spectrum of lucidity. This is based on the degrees of awareness within the dream, ranging from a suspicion that we might be dreaming to fully conscious reflective awareness.

I've identified four main levels on the spectrum, although this is a very basic system of categorization and it's not necessary to stick to it rigidly. Our progress along the spectrum isn't always a linear one either, and although Level 1 may often lead to Level 2 and so on, it is also common to find ourselves at Level 3 or 4 straightaway, thanks to a sudden burst of awareness.

Level 1: Pre-lucid

'Pre-lucid' is a term coined by lucid dream researcher Celia Green to describe the state of mind in which we critically question the reality of the dream. Although this experience can lead straight to lucidity, it's often a state that beginners may visit frustratingly frequently without becoming lucid.

In the pre-lucid state, suspicions arise that we might be dreaming, usually after we have become aware of some bizarre dream anomaly. For example, we are pre-lucid if we find ourselves in a dream thinking, *Hang on, I don't usually go out in public in my underwear... Could I be dreaming?*

Level 2: Semi-lucid

Here we experience the 'Aha!' moment of lucid awareness but then slip back and forth between lucidity and non-lucidity. We may be lucid one moment, then become distracted by the dream and slip back into non-lucidity. Alternatively, 'semi-lucid' can describe the state of lucidity in which we know that we are dreaming but simply allow the dream to play out without any interaction or intervention of any kind.

More commonly, the initial 'lucidity flash' can be so exciting that we wake ourselves up. *Hang on, I don't usually go out in public in my underwear... Could I be dreaming?* soon becomes *Oh, wow! I actually am dreaming! This is so cool! I can't wait to try to...* and then we find ourselves awake in our bed. In fact, for some beginners, this initial over-excitability means that their first few lucid dreams may only last a matter of seconds before they wake up. (We'll look at ways to avoid this in Part II.)

Level 3: Fully Lucid

This is the state of fully conscious reflective awareness within the dream, coupled with volitional interaction with the dreamscape and dream characters. We can now co-create the dream at will.

Here we are fully aware that we're dreaming and can begin to influence the dreamscape and narrative of the dream by engaging in whatever activity we want to do. With full lucidity, we can maintain awareness for the entirety of the dream period, which may be an hour or more in length.

Many believe this is the highest possible level of lucidity. I disagree – there is a deeper level.

Level 4: Super-lucid

This is a term borrowed from Robert Waggoner to describe the state in which we have a level of awareness that surpasses full lucidity, due to an experience of partial non-dual awareness.

What does this mean? The fundamental difference between 'fully lucid' and 'super-lucid' rests on a subtle but profound shift of perception. Most of us experiencing a fully lucid dream will interact with the dream as if it is waking reality. For example, we might use a door to get from one room to another or fly through the air to travel to a new place. In a super-lucid dream, however, we'll just walk straight through the wall or instantly appear somewhere at will rather than travel there. While super-lucid, we base all our actions upon the realization that everything in the dream is a creation of the mind, without slipping back into the dualistic interactions of lower-level full lucidity.*

---

* A super-lucid dream is, for many people, an experience approaching non-dual awareness in which the clarity of mind is so strong that it may shatter the dreamer's sense of self.

Witnessing Dream

This type of dream falls within the lucidity spectrum but doesn't quite fit into any of the four levels described previously. We experience a witnessing dream from a gentle non-preferential perspective, fully aware that we are dreaming but without any desire to influence or interact with the dream. Instead we allow it to unfold on its own, often as though we are watching the dream on a movie screen.

Witnessing dreams can happen spontaneously, but are a common product of prolonged periods of meditation – the meditator effectively carries the daytime's quiet non-preferential mindfulness into the night.*

•••

Don't worry too much about the different levels of lucidity. I've included the lucidity spectrum here more to explore the nature of lucidity than to make it a cornerstone of the practice.

Does Lucid Dreaming Mean We're Controlling Our Dreams?

Many books and websites promise the ability to 'control your dreams through lucid dreaming', but this is an ill-advised – and arguably impossible – aim. Although it's true that with training an advanced practitioner can gain a remarkable level of volitional influence over many aspects of their subjective experience, there is always a much larger aspect of mind creating and controlling the majority of the dream.

---

* Rubin Naiman, PhD, comments in his *Yoga of Sleep* audiobook that meditators are more likely to have spontaneous awareness during sleep because they are accessing similar states of consciousness during their meditation.

Once lucid, it is of course natural to want to exert our will. One of the most popular lucid dream activities seems to be flying, so let's work with that example. Say you become lucid and choose to fly into the sky. Arms outstretched like Superman and you're off. You're controlling the dream, right? Wrong.

Even in a lucid dream in which you're flying through the air, controlling your elevation and velocity at will, there is still a much larger aspect of mind creating and managing the dream landscape that you're flying over and the dream sky that you're flying in. Did you choose to have those dream characters walking the streets below you? You may be controlling your subjective experience of the localized dreamscape, but there is something much more powerful directing everything else.

Waggoner says, 'No sailor controls the sea. Similarly, no lucid dreamer controls the dream.'[9] A sailor controls their boat, but it would be an arrogant sailor who believed that they were controlling the awesome power of the sea, and it's just the same with our dreams.

I didn't always believe this, though. Through a lot of intensive training in my 20s, I once reached a level of lucidity in which I would change the entire dreamscape just because I could, silence dream characters to show them I was boss and forcefully reject new lines of narrative in favour of my own. I thought that finally, after years of practice, I had gained full control over my dreams, but in fact I was disregarding the music of the dreaming mind and forcefully dancing to my own beat, totally out of synch with what the dream was trying to offer. These attempts would invariably lead to a loving but firm slap from the motherly dreaming mind, either through an inexplicable loss of lucid control or a bombardment of nightmarish shadow material.

Once I began to relinquish the excessive control I had been exercising, something strange happened – I started to have more volitional influence within my lucid dreams, not less. It was as if once

I had shifted my motivation from *control* to *co-creation*, the dreaming mind responded positively by giving me more lucid capacity.

A sailor may grow to know the sea so well that he sails *as if* he were in control. So, too, we can come to sail upon the ocean of our dreaming mind.

Are We Messing with the Unconscious?

Another concern we should address at the outset is the fear that by lucid dreaming we may somehow be interfering with the integrity of the unconscious by bringing awareness into an area of our mind that normally seems to function autonomously. Thankfully, this fear is groundless.

Rather than lucid dreaming polluting the pure message from the deeper part of ourselves, it actually allows that message to be heeded more easily, which I believe is exactly what the unconscious mind wants. The unconscious actually enjoys lucidity, because finally a line of direct communication is being set up between it and the conscious mind, and it 'takes joy in dealing with greater awareness and greater consciousness'.[10] Finally, it can talk to us face to face.

With every dream, the unconscious mind is offering us a hand of friendship. But far too often this is an offering we ignore, either by not remembering our dreams or by failing to acknowledge their value. Once we become lucid within the dream, however, we are extending the hand of friendship towards the unconscious mind and finally making friends with it.

As Rob Preece says in *The Psychology of Buddhist Tantra*, 'When we are willing to take the psyche seriously, and listen to its symbolic expression, we can gain greater clarity and insight into the forces that influence us. We will no longer be victims of the unconscious.'[11]

This is one of the core benefits of lucid dreaming: making friends with ourselves. We don't get lucid so we can try to control the unconscious mind or boss it about, we get lucid so that we can make friends with it, commune with it and finally start listening to it.

As with any friendship, we have to learn to accept our new friend on equal terms, not censoring or arguing with them, but listening to them with an open heart. This is the most important friendship we may ever have, and it is a friendship that will spill over into our waking state, too, in sudden bursts of creativity or spontaneous insights that let us know our new friend is always with us – even when we're not dreaming.

Although this friendship may be on equal terms, the unconscious has been running the dream state for much longer than we've been trying to have intentional lucid dreams, and so it will always be the stronger force. We're not talking about taking some drug that compels the unconscious mind to accommodate lucid awareness, but a process by which the dreaming mind opens the door and allows lucidity into its domain.* This means that if it doesn't like what we're doing in the lucid dream, it will simply block our attempts to do whatever it is, so to think that we can 'mess with the unconscious' just because we are lucid is to ascribe an inflated degree of influence to our conscious mind.

Can Everyone Do It?

The good news is that everybody can learn to lucid dream. In fact, we don't even really need to learn, we just need to remember.

Picasso once said, 'Every child is born an artist; the adult's job is to remember how,' and it seems to be the same with lucid dreaming.

A 1998 study called 'Age-dependent dreaming' reported that about 30 per cent of adolescents from 14 to 17 experienced lucid dreams once or twice a week,[12] having between 50–100 spontaneous

---

* We have about five dream periods each night, so even if we have a lucid dream every night, there are still four other dream periods in which our unconscious mind can run wild and free.

lucid dreams per year – a percentage that is much higher than that reported by adults.

A study of British schoolchildren conducted by Swansea University[13] found that lucid dreaming was common in children, with 43.5 per cent of the 6-to-18-year-olds surveyed having had at least one lucid dream, and a 2012 study[14] from Harvard Medical School professor Allan Hobson and Ursula Voss found that lucid dreaming was quite pronounced in young children and even proposed a link between the natural occurrence of lucid dreaming and brain maturation.

Charlie says

'Parents might be interested to know that a 2006 study[15] found a direct correlation between video-gaming and lucid dream frequency, while a 2012 study[16] showed an increase in lucid dreaming among children who read fantasy fiction. I will leave it to individual parents to decide which of the two activities to encourage!'

The fact that lucid dreaming comes factory-installed tells us two crucial things. First, that you have almost certainly had dozens of lucid dreams before, whether you remember them or not, and second that you don't need to *learn* to lucid dream, you need to *remember*. One of the best ways to remember is to reconnect with the part of yourself that first lucidly dreamed: your inner child (*in Chapter 7 we'll learn how*).

My personal theory on why children have so many spontaneous lucid dreams is connected to creativity. Most children are naturally right-brain dominant, meaning they are attuned to the creative, imaginative, intuitive side of their brain. But as they grow up, they switch sides to the more logical, calculating, left-brain dominance of adulthood. Dreaming is an almost entirely right-brain activity, so it seems that once we lose our connection to the creativity of our brain's right hemisphere, we also lose our connection to our dreams – and our natural ability to become lucid within them. In short, we forget how to lucid dream when we forget how to be children. Artistic adults such as actors, musicians and artists, however, often retain their right-brain inclination, which is why they seem to have spontaneous lucid dreams more often than other people.

So, lucid dreaming is a perfectly natural state of mind and we can regain it. The Buddha once said, 'It doesn't matter how long you have forgotten, only how soon you remember.' So don't worry how long it has been since you last had a lucid dream, let's just concentrate on remembering how to do it again. The fact is, if you dream, you can lucid dream – it just takes some practice.

Throughout this book I quote research studies from many different sleep laboratories, but the best 'sleep lab' we have is the one in our own bed, a lab to which we have access every night.

As a teenager, the free accessibility of lucid dreaming was one of its real selling points for me. There was no equipment to be bought, no initiation to be done, no club to join. The only commodities required were sleep and determination. And the great thing about dream work, compared to other mind-training tools, is that hardly a 24-hour period goes by without the opportunity to practise. Whether you are a nightshift worker snoozing in the afternoon, a student sleeping till lunchtime or a pensioner dozing during the day, there is always time for lucid dreaming.

As with all skills, some people may find it easier than others. It seems that having two X chromosomes can help, as females report more lucid dreams and have better dream recall than males, but essentially lucid dreaming is open to everyone. Teenagers and people under the age of 30 have longer dream periods and thus slightly more opportunity to practise, but unless you have a strong motivation to become lucid, it doesn't matter how much dream time you have. I've taught everyone from 10-year-olds to 80-year-olds, and the defining characteristic of success is motivation, not age.

A lot of the lucid dreaming workshops and retreats that I run take place at Buddhist centres and I have found that practising meditators have much more stability in their lucid dreams than non-meditators. This is because the stability of mindful awareness during the day directly translates into the stability of awareness during dreams.

If meditation seems a bit too static for you, then it seems that getting down on the dance floor might work just as well. Before teaching lucid dreaming, I spent many years working in the world of professional breakdancing, and I noticed that many of my dancer friends found lucid dreaming remarkably easy. Was it all that spinning on their head that did it? Perhaps dream researcher Jayne Gackenbach says that due to the link between the vestibular system of balance found in the inner ear and the production of eye movements during dreams, people who have good physical body balance (such as breakdancers) are often good at lucid dreaming.[17] Another finding Gackenbach came up with is one of my personal favourites: apparently, lucid dreamers are 'often people who lean towards an androgynous temperament and those who are willing to take internal risks such as trying shamanic drumming'.[18] Who knew?

New research, which we'll explore later, has shown that engaging in 'flow-state' activities can increase the frequency of lucid dreams. This might explain the link to both dancing and drumming, as flow states are reached when you're giving your fullest attention to an activity or task that you are singularly focused on and totally immersed in. The mind's usual chatter begins to fade away, placing you in a non-distracted state often referred to as being 'in the zone'. People who are in that state a lot, such as dancers, musicians, rock-climbers and athletes, tend to have more lucid dreams.

So it seems that if you are an artistic, mindful, breakdancing female shamanic-drumming teenager who does lots of flow-state activities, you might find lucid dreaming a bit easier than the rest of us. But if you are none of the above, not to worry – we can all learn how to lucid dream. And in Part II I'll show you how.

CHAPTER 2
THE SCIENCE OF LUCIDITY

*'The history of the world is none other than the
progress of the consciousness of freedom.'*

Hegel

It's just gone 8 a.m. on a rainy spring morning at Hull University in 1975. Psychologist Keith Hearne is hunched over a recording apparatus charting the eye movements, muscle tone and EEG brain activity of his sleeping subject, a 37-year-old lucid dreamer named Alan Worsley. Although he doesn't know it yet, Worsley is about to make history.

When Hearne decided to tackle the scientific verification of lucid dreaming, the concept was still scoffed at by the scientific community as being a 'paradoxical impossibility'. Regardless of thousands of years of first-hand reports and an entire arena of Buddhist teachings on the subject, most sleep and dream researchers considered the idea of conscious awareness within dreams a flaky New Age delusion.

Hearne's contemporaries realized that the only way to verify lucid dreaming scientifically would be to get data that proved two things simultaneously: first, that the dreamer was dreaming and not partially awake; second, that the dreamer was consciously signalling to the outside world from within the dream world. But how to send such a signal without waking up? During dreaming sleep the body is paralysed – with the exception of the respiratory system and the eyes. Hearne had a hunch that the eyes could be used to send that all-important signal.

Before falling asleep, Worsley was instructed to try to become lucid and then engage in a set of smooth horizontal eye movements (very different from the random flitting and rolling of REM sleep). These signals would then be picked up by the eye-movement recorders in the lab, while the EEG machine would keep track of his brain activity.

The night passed with little success, but in the final hour of Worsley's sleep cycle his periods of REM became more frequent. Hearne had been watching Worsley dreaming for about half an hour when something remarkable happened.

'Suddenly, out of the jumbled, senseless tos and fros of the two eye-movement recording channels, a regular set of large zig-zags appeared on the chart,' Hearne recalls in his book *Dream Machine*. 'Instantly I was alert and felt the greatest exhilaration upon realizing that I was observing the first ever deliberate signals sent from within the dream to the outside world.'[1] The 'impossible' had finally been proved.

Around the same time that Hearne was pioneering the scientific verification of lucid dreaming in the UK, in the USA a bright young lucid dreamer was starting work on his PhD in psychophysiology at Stanford University in California. This prodigal dreamer was Stephen LaBerge, a name that would become synonymous with lucid dreaming across the globe. Working at Stanford, LaBerge set out to prove the existence of lucid dreaming for the first time in history – or so he thought.

How could he not have known about Hearne's results? Although Hearne did deliver a paper to a conference on behavioural sciences in 1977, then published his PhD thesis a

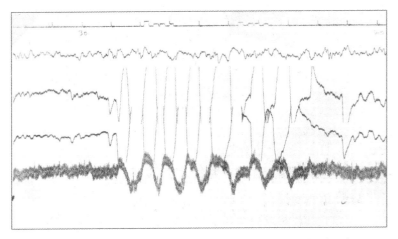

The first-ever recorded ocular signals from a person in a lucid dream. The two central bands above show the movement records for the left and right eyes. We can clearly see just how definite the eye-movement signals were when compared to the jittery, short waves of rapid eye movement that both precede and follow them.

year later, 'the scientific establishment resisted accepting his results'.[2] The upshot was that his proof was simply never widely circulated, peer-reviewed or disseminated across the Atlantic. When LaBerge finally got similar results using similar methods, he naturally believed that he had broken new ground. This proved a useful illusion, as it fed his determination to spread the news when all the top journals (including the esteemed *Science*) refused to publish his research. Eventually, in 1981, a lesser-known scientific journal, *Perceptual and Motor Skills*, published his findings.[3] This, along with a primetime lecture spot at the Association for the Psycho-physiological Study of Sleep's annual conference, was the start of an epic career that would make LaBerge the pioneer of lucid dreaming in the West.

LaBerge's passion for the subject and his notable aptitude both for lucid dreaming and for teaching it to others have relegated much of Hearne's impeccable research to a footnote in the history books. However, without LaBerge's tireless work over the last four decades in both the public and scientific spheres, lucid dreaming books might still be in the New Age section. We would do well to doff our hats to both Hearne and LaBerge.

Beyond the Imagination

Since those initial experiments in the days of disco, scientific research into lucid dreaming has thrown up scores of weird and wonderful new discoveries, with one conclusion and its implications standing out from the rest.

Using EEG machines, eye-movement and muscle-tone monitors in experiments that involved activities like singing* and mental arithmetic within the lucid dream state, it was discovered that lucid dream actions elicited exactly the same neurological responses as actions performed while awake.

Further research found that holding your breath, estimating time (lucid dream time and waking time feeling roughly the same) and even practising sports in a lucid dream all elicit the exact same brain responses as when awake.

In fact we have over 40 years' worth of sport science studies that pretty much all conclude that people who intentionally practise their athletic discipline in their lucid dreams actually get better at it in the waking state.

A 2011 study at Heidelberg University, Germany, and the University of Bern, Switzerland, concluded that: 'Lucid dreams have a great potential for athletes to use as a training method because

---

* Interestingly, the first song to be sung in the lucid dream state by LaBerge's research team was 'Life is but a Dream'.

lucid dreaming mimics a perfect simulation of the real world... without the limitations of reality.'[4]

A 2018 study[5] that I actually participated in found that '81.3% of participants reported positive effects of lucid dream martial arts training' on their waking-state performance. Athletes have been using waking-state visualization to improve their performance for decades, though, right? Yes, but, as the chief researcher of one of the lucid dream studies said, 'Training in a lucid dream can produce better results than visualized training in the waking state, because in the lucid dream you experience your movements in a far more realistic way.'[6]

Other researchers agree and say that the main downside of waking visualization is that 'if the mental imagery technique is performed inadequately, without sufficient attention, subsequent gains in motor performance will be substandard'.[7] Lucid dreaming, however, solves this problem, because it is the most complete visualization possible and allows for the most complete realization of the technique.

It's not just motor skills that can be honed through the strength of our imagination – we can actually strengthen our muscles, too.[8] Researchers at the Cleveland Clinic Foundation in 2004 asked a group of people to imagine lifting weights with their arms for 15 minutes a day, five days a week, for 12 weeks. At the end of their study, they concluded: 'Subjects who imagined lifting heavy weights with their arms increased their bicep strength by 13.5% on average and the gain in strength lasted for three months after they stopped the mental exercise regime.'[9]

If those gains in muscle strength were made through simple waking visualization, just imagine what gains could be made in the complete visualization of the lucid dream state. So, next time you're in a lucid dream, try doing a few press-ups – it might give you gains you've only ever dreamed of.

Bigger Brains

It's not only your muscles that can get bigger through lucid dreaming, it's also your brain. It turns out that lucid dreaming not only has the potential to rewire our brain but to actually change its physical structure.

In 2015 a study from the Max Planck Institute of Psychiatry published in the *Journal of Neuroscience* found that 'People who were better at lucid dreaming also showed higher levels of activity in the anterior prefrontal cortex'[10] and that because of this, lucid dreamers had 'greater grey matter volume in this part of the brain – thus making this part of the brain actually larger'.[11]

Was there any actual benefit to this increase in brain volume, though? Yes, both this study and a previous one show that it gives lucid dreamers higher levels of creative lateral thinking in the waking state and makes them able to 'solve significantly more insight problems than non-lucid dreamers'.[12]

Charlie says

'Yup, although it sounds like click bait, this means that we can honestly say that lucid dreaming gives you a bigger brain! It's just one of the many mindboggling takeaways of lucid dreaming.'

With so much new lucid dream science being published in the last 10 years (more than in the last 50 put together, actually), I find myself being constrained by page count rather than content, but I'd be missing a trick if I didn't share this final study.

In 2021, scientists from four different laboratories, including Northwestern University in Chicago, proved for the first time ever that it was possible to engage not only communication from the dream state to the waking state (as Hearne and Worsley had done), but actually from the waking state to the dream state and back again.[13]

Scientists worked with 36 participants to see if it was possible for lucid dreamers to hear and understand questions sent from the waking state and then communicate an answer back to the waking state while they were still asleep. How did they do this?

The participants fell asleep in the laboratory hooked up to all sorts of brain scanners to indicate when they were dreaming. Once a dreamer became lucid, they would communicate with the scientists in the lab by flicking their eyes in a prearranged pattern, *à la* Hearne and Worsley.

The scientists then communicated with the sleeping subject through a microphone hooked up to a set of headphones that they were wearing and asked them questions, which then entered the dream while the subject was still asleep. The scientists asked maths questions: things like eight minus six, for example. To answer the questions, the dreamers used the eye signals again, flicking their eyes Morse-code-style to communicate the answer.

That process in itself was mind-blowing, but it was the description of how the voice of the scientist was incorporated into the dream that really struck me. For one dreamer, it came through a car radio; for another, it was the 'voice of God' from the sky; and for another, it was like a narrator in a movie.

This kind of complex two-way communication from the waking state to the lucid dream opens up huge possibilities. The lead researcher of the study from Northwestern University said that she hoped this technique could be used therapeutically in the future to help people better deal with trauma, anxiety and depression. Later on we dedicate whole chapters to the potential of using lucid dreaming to treat PTSD, trauma and nightmares, and there's a lot of science to back this up, too. In fact, a 2019 scientific review of more than 10 different papers on Lucid Dream Therapy (yup, it's a thing) concluded that lucid dreaming can 'aid in the treatment of patients with nightmares through minimizing their frequency, intensity and level of psychological distress'.[14]

Charlie says

'I've taught lucid dreaming to many highly traumatized populations, and the thought that one day I might be able to directly communicate with them while they are inside a lucid nightmare, for example, and help guide them to face their fear or to integrate their trauma in real time would truly be a dream come true.'

These scientific studies open up a whole arena for psychological healing and growth. We can *learn* in lucid dreams. We can change our brain in lucid dreams. We can learn to use the lucid dream state not just as a rehearsal space for waking life, but as a laboratory of transformation that allows us to make lasting changes to our mind while we sleep.

Now that we know about the science of lucid dreaming, let's look at how this practice can actually benefit us in everyday life. In what ways might we want to rewire our brain? Which aspects of our mind might we want to explore? How can lucid dreaming make us happier and healthier? Let's find out.

CHAPTER 3

THE PSYCHOLOGICAL BENEFITS OF LUCID DREAMING

*'There is no better way to show the mind
how our concept of reality can be blown away
than through practising lucid dreaming.'*

Rob Nairn[1]

One of the main changes to the way I have been teaching since the first edition of this book has been the full embrace of the idea that the 'why' is more important than the 'how'.

We will of course learn 'how' to lucid dream later on, but before that it's vital we explore 'why' we're doing it. Why do you want to have lucid dreams? It takes time and effort, so unless you have a very good reason why you want to become lucid, you may find that the effort outweighs the perceived reward.

However, if you perceive the reward of lucid dreaming as anything less than life-changing, then you simply haven't understood its full potential. I've seen people heal post-traumatic stress disorder, have spiritual breakthroughs, integrate their depression, remedy physical ailments, let go of grief, get better at sports and even integrate childhood trauma, all through lucid dreaming.

These weren't Buddhist monks or special people, but everyday people like you and me who discovered one of the most powerful self-development tools in existence and used it to radically alter their lives.

So, let's do a deep dive into the 'why' of lucid dreaming.

Accessing the Library

Our unconscious mind holds a wealth of information about ourselves and the world around us. This knowledge can rarely be accessed in the waking state, but in a lucid dream we are given the keys to the library and admission to the deepest recesses of the most ancient and reserved sections, in which we can reference every experience that we have ever had: the literal biography of our lives, and of previous ones, too.*

According to the well-known hypnotherapy expert Valerie Austin, 'everything we have ever done, said, heard, smelled or seen is stored away in the subconscious'[2]** and hypnosis 'allows us access to this data straight from the subconscious without being edited by our rational conscious mind'.[3] A very similar process occurs during lucid dreaming, but the amount of data that we can access is much, much larger.

Once we have the keys to the library, answers to questions that we may spend hours of talking therapy trying to discover (such as 'What is my greatest fear?' or 'What is the source of my depression?') become accessible to us.

---

* For Swiss psychiatrist Carl Jung, certain dream content was even transpersonal, sourced from a vast storehouse of ancient human experience containing themes and images found cross-culturally throughout history. This observation led to his concept of the 'collective unconscious' and he argued that dream symbols could also point beyond the personal and into the realm of this depository of human experience.

** Many people use 'subconscious' and 'unconscious' interchangeably, but I tend to use the term 'unconscious' when dealing with dreams, as this was the term that both Freud and Jung used.

Just as we can access the information already in the library, we can also add to its shelves. If, when we become lucid, we plant the seed of a beneficial idea or suggestion in the fertile soil of the unconscious, it penetrates the deepest levels of our mind and affects our waking state in a tangible fashion. By calling out beneficial statements of intent while in the lucid dream or engaging in new habit patterns such as generosity or fearlessness, we can write new ideas and modes of behaviour into the very code of our being. Just as we can rewire our brain, we can also recode our psyche.

Our unconscious mind is actually trying to communicate with us every time we dream, lucidly or not. The library of knowledge that resides in our dreaming mind is open to us every time we sleep and its content will be presented to us whether we're conscious of it or not. This is why it's good to be interested in all our dreams, not just the lucid ones: by being more mindful of our dreams, we extend a hand of friendship to our deepest parts. Dreaming is the most intimate relationship that we have with ourselves, and every night our unconscious mind opens a window into our psyche through a narrative of symbols and imagery.

In the words of Marc Barasch, author of *Healing Dreams*:

> *Our dreams disturb us because they refuse to pander to our fondest notions of ourselves. The closer one looks, the more they seem to insist upon a challenging proposition: You must live truthfully. Right now. And always. Few forces in life present, with an equal sense of inevitability, the bare-knuckle facts of who we are, and the demands of what we might become.*[4]

All too often these are communications that we either ignore or forget. But by learning how to appreciate and engage our dream world by simply bringing more mindfulness into our dreams and reflecting on them, let alone practising lucid dreaming, we begin to access the library and unlock its wisdom.

Healing the Inner Child

One of the most powerful benefits of lucid dreaming that I've witnessed in both myself and my clients over the past 10 years has been healing the inner child.

Time magazine published an article in their April 2023 edition titled 'Why is everyone working on their inner child?',[5] so it seems as if the benefits of this deep work are finally making it into the mainstream.

Dr Charles Whitfield, author of *Healing the Child Within*, tells us that the concept of the inner child has been around for over 2,000 years, but in the West it was the psychiatrist Carl Jung who popularized it as the archetypal representation of our childhood experiences (both harmful and helpful).

Jung believed that we all had an inner child, a part of ourselves forever connected to both our past childhood experiences and our present childlike energy, or lack of it. Our inner child is the current expression of our connection to playfulness, joy and innocence and also the summation of all of our actual childhood experiences and the unmet needs of the idealized child that we hoped we might be.

Charlie says

'Childlike but not childish is a crucial distinction to make between the healthy inner child and the wounded one. In adulthood, we experience the healthy aspects of the inner child whenever we feel moments of childlike joy and experience the wounded aspects whenever we are triggered into childish reactivity.'

Mexican Toltec teacher Don Miguel Ruiz says that the inner child is expressed when you are 'having fun or being playful, when you feel happy when you are painting, or writing poetry, or playing the piano, or expressing yourself freely in some way. These are often the happiest moments of your life... when you are childlike.'6

Due to it being the dominant internal archetype of our childhood, when traumatic childhood experiences negatively affect us, it is our inner child that may carry these wounds.

A wounded inner child leads not only to an inability to fully connect to our inner joy, but also to acting out childhood patterns in our adult life. We have all had experiences of never quite being loved the way we needed as a child, and most of us would agree that childhood experiences leave an almost indelible mark on the psyche and, although often seemingly forgotten, still impact us in adulthood.

Without implying that everyone has childhood trauma, we can say for sure that everyone has had a childhood with tough moments: feelings of dependency, helplessness, frustration and vulnerability. By healing our inner child, we begin the process of reparenting ourselves and of creating the conditions of safety and love that will allow us to tap into the authentic joy and wisdom of our healthy inner child.

Esteemed psychotherapist David Richo, PhD, believes that healing the inner child is 'of paramount importance for our psychological health and well-being' and that to fully step into adulthood, we must befriend, heal and empower our inner child.

Inner child healing is about doing the work that was denied to us as children and using our present-state resources to heal our childhood wounds. Lucid dreaming provides us with the perfect space to do this, because we can, in the form of our capable and well-resourced adult selves, literally meet, hug, comfort and even dialogue with a personification of our inner child. (In Chapter 7 we will learn exactly how to do that, but if you can't wait until then, check out my own inner child healing in Dream 20 on page 284.)

Curing Depression

In 2021 I received an email titled: 'I cured depression thanks to lucid dreaming.' Although a University of Heidelberg study concluded that 'Lucid dream work may be an effective treatment for mental health issues, including clinical depression,'[7] it was with a hint of scepticism that I opened the email. In it, Matt Humphreys, a 31-year-old graphic designer from the UK, explained how he had cured himself of 10 years of treatment-resistant depression through lucid dreaming.

After years of CBT, anti-depressants and, in his words, 'going from shrink to shrink' with no success, he saw some of my YouTube videos and then read one of my books and decided that he would try to use lucid dreaming to heal his depression.

When he became lucid, he remembered his intention and called out to the dream, 'Why am I always so depressed? Show me the source of my depression.'

The dream responded by presenting him with his grandmother, who had died from Alzheimer's disease when he was a child. What happened next was quite amazing, so I'll let Matt tell it in his own words:

> Obviously I hadn't seen her since she had died, so it was a shock to see her in the lucid dream. She was scared. She was shaking. Looked really ill. I thought: How is my dead nan the reason why I'm so depressed? And then I had a light-bulb moment and suddenly realized: Yes! I felt so guilty about her death. I never wanted to visit her, or speak to her, it was a chore. The old people's home was smelly and I never wanted to go. I was a kid, I hated it. Then when she died, I felt so guilty.
>
> As soon as I realized this in the lucid dream, my grandmother physically changed — as if my realization made her change. She suddenly looked healthy, how she had looked before the Alzheimer's.

Then I remembered what you said in your videos and I hugged her. It felt incredible, just total bliss. A weight lifted from my shoulders – I could just feel it draining away. The hug felt like it lasted forever, but it was probably only a few seconds.

Then I woke up, beaming! It took a couple of days, though, for me to actually realize that the cloud of depression had gone. It had totally changed. That one lucid dream did more for me than years of medication and CBT.

It's been almost three years now and Matt is still depression-free. In fact, his quotes are taken not only from that 2021 email, but also from a talk that I gave recently in London at which Matt came up on stage to share his story.

What really impressed me about Matt's story is how it does actually fit within the model of childhood trauma integration in which it is believed that if we can find the 'original wound' (usually a painful childhood experience), then healing can occur at a very deep level, because we have found the source of the river, the root cause.

Charlie says

'A year or so after our first contact I received another unexpected email – from Matt's dad this time! He wrote: "Matt today is a completely different person – his stress and anxiety have gone, he takes life in his stride, is happily married and has settled down. This lucid dreaming is powerful stuff. Matt has been showing me how to do it too!"'

Healing the Body

Many people believe in the potential for physical healing through visualization, such as the method in which patients imagine their body's immune system healing diseased cells in the form of coloured light. Studies have shown that this kind of visualized healing can help to reduce stress, enhance the immune system and lessen pain[8] in many patients. These techniques are dependent upon our ability to visualize, however – something not all of us find so easy.

In a lucid dream, the playing field is levelled, because a lucid dream is the most vivid and complete visualization we can experience. Applying those healing techniques within a lucid dream may prove far more effective than any visualization done in the waking state.* This is well established in the Tibetan Buddhist teachings, which say that while lucid, 'the power of the mind is heightened', making visualized healing 'far more powerful than simply visualizing in the waking state'.[9] I personally know of lucid dreamers either healing or drastically reducing the symptoms of everything from knee problems to kidney disease to allergic rhinitis, and there are lots more examples in Robert Waggoner's book *Lucid Dreaming: Gateway to the Inner Self* to corroborate this. I myself have healed ear infections and torn ligaments through visualized healing in lucid dreams. (*In Chapter 7 we will look at exactly how to engage physical healing in lucid dreams.*)

Although at the time of writing we have no scientific studies to back up these purely anecdotal claims, much of the initial scepticism that people may have about the potential for lucid dream healing can be assuaged by learning about the placebo effect, a phenomenon that Professor Richard Wiseman from University of Hertfordshire says has been shown to account for a staggering 60–90 per cent of the effectiveness of some medical drugs.[10]

A placebo effect study run by Professor Wiseman showed that test subjects who were served drinks that tasted and smelled identical to alcoholic drinks but were actually alcohol-free displayed

---

* For a great example of physical healing through a lucid dream, see Dream 16, page 279.

signs not only of physical inebriation, but of mental inebriation too. He said that 'just believing that they had been drinking alcohol was enough to convince their brains and bodies to behave in a drunk way'.[11]

The epidemiologist Dr Ben Goldacre, a man whose mission is to combat the dissemination of misleading scientific data, agrees that although the placebo effect is 'an outrageous and ridiculous phenomenon, it is true. For some aliments, two sugar pills a day is the most effective treatment available. It's all about our beliefs and expectations.'[12]

So for those who cry, 'It's just the placebo effect!' when presented with stories of lucid dream healing, I reply, 'Yes, it may well be. And yet, the healing still occurs.'

Charlie says

'The Tibetan Buddhist master Namkhai Norbu Rinpoche used to teach a particular practice to treat cancer that entailed visualizing a tiny red-hot garuda (a mythological bird) at the location of the cancer and imagining it burning up cancer cells. It was said that to do this in a lucid dream greatly enhanced its effectiveness.'

There is also the potential to heal phobias within the lucid dream state. Scared of spiders? Use the lucid dream to touch a spider or hold one in your hand, engaging with it in the knowledge that it isn't real, it's just a mental projection. This new fearless engagement with the object of the phobia will leave a neurological pathway in the brain that may be activated in the waking state, too, thus paving the way to curing the phobia for good.

Remember that when we become lucid, we aren't just contacting the unconscious mind, as in hypnosis, but are actually submerged in its deepest depths, so if, once lucid, we call out an affirmation to integrate our fear of heights (for example, 'I feel safe and secure at all heights'), this suggestion might work far more powerfully that hypnosis alone.

As for addictions, these can be worked on in exactly the same way as you would in hypnotherapy, by offering the unconscious mind a beneficial suggestion pertaining to altering an addictive behaviour pattern, or, as Antonio, a case study in my second book, *Lucid Dreaming Made Easy*, did, by meeting a personification of your brain and asking it to help curb the addiction. (That one lucid dream ended Antonio's years of nicotine addiction.)

Transforming Nightmares

When I was 17, I had an accidental LSD overdose and near-death experience, which was terrifying and led to months of nightmares. At the time I had just read one of my first lucid dreaming books and remembered the section on using lucidity to heal nightmares, but whenever I got lucid within these recurrent nightmares I was so consumed by fear and dread that I usually just ended up yelling, 'Wake up! I want to wake up!' Unfortunately, this just happens to be the most effective way of ensuring that a nightmare recurs, because in no way does it resolve or heal the psychological trauma fuelling it.

An unfinished nightmare is like an unfinished therapy session, and because your mind loves you and is always striving for homeostasis, it tries to finish the therapy session by giving you the same or a similar nightmare again. So, if you are ever lucky enough to find yourself lucid in a nightmare, don't try to wake up. Stay in it if you can.

The simple act of choosing to stay in a nightmare is such an empowering statement of your intent to finally witness and integrate your trauma that, in and of itself, it will often lead to the full cessation of nightmares.

And that's pretty much what happened with me when I was 17. One night I finally decided I'd had enough. I set a strong threefold motivation: to intentionally invoke the nightmare, to become lucid within it and to face the source of the trauma.

That very night the nightmare came and the little bald-headed dwarf who had somehow come to represent the trauma appeared as usual, signifying insanity and death. But this time I recognized that I was dreaming, and as he approached me, I finally turned to face him. Rather than run away, I yelled at him: 'OK, I get it! I see now! I see! Just fuck off!'

Of course, I now know that I could have sent him love or hugged him, but the act of standing my ground and setting my boundaries seems to work just as well in this instance. Suddenly the dwarf's face changed and then the entire dreamscape changed into a 17-year-old's vision of paradise – in this case, bikini-clad girls dancing on top of a skate ramp while people were skateboarding and drinking cocktails in the sun. Not very subtle, but the best my teenage mind could muster.

That was the last time I ever had that nightmare. Four months of post-traumatic stress cured by one lucid dream. It was then that I realized the huge potential of lucid dreaming.

Charlie says

'Having the courage to stand your ground and say, "This is all just a dream. This is my mind. I am safe. My body is asleep in bed, I am not back in that traumatic event, I am just dreaming about it" is so dramatically different from how we usually relate to our trauma that it can lead to similarly dramatic levels of integration.'

Chapters 10 and 11 are dedicated to treating nightmares and PTSD trauma through lucid dreaming, but for now, let's just say that if you can experience a nightmare with full lucidity, you have a powerful opportunity for trauma resolution and psychological integration, which is likely to lead to the cessation of the nightmares.

Could this mean there may be a time in the future when doctors will give nightmare sufferers a prescription for lucid dream training rather than a prescription for medication? I'm working on it, but for now we can but dream.

Integrating the Shadow

The concept of the shadow is found within almost every culture and spiritual tradition the world over, but it was first popularized in the West by the legendary Swiss psychiatrist Carl Jung.

The shadow is our dark side, but not dark as in 'negative' or 'malign', rather dark ·as in 'not yet illuminated'. It comprises everything within us that we don't want to face. That is, everything, both seemingly harmful and potentially enlightening – all that we have rejected, denied, disowned or repressed.*

We hide the traits we don't like about ourselves from the world and from ourselves. We shove them into the recesses of our mind, where they gather, and from where they occasionally erupt, or spill forth when our guard is dropped. Preferring to remain unaware of our own shadow aspects, we find they become a dangerous influence, often lurking just beneath the surface. Jung said, 'Everyone carries a shadow, and the less it is embodied in the individual's conscious life, the darker and denser it is.'[13]

Anything that we deem unacceptable and deny within ourselves forms the shadow, but it's crucial to understand that the shadow is not evil or bad, it's simply the parts of ourselves that seem

---

* A young boy who has been caught dancing by his macho father and been chastised for it may well repress his inner dancer, and so his shadow might contain the very positive potential of creativity and dance. This is what makes up what is known as the golden shadow.

incompatible with who we think we are. Jung said that the shadow was 90 per cent pure gold. He knew that it was just as full of our unexpressed talents and spiritual power as it was of our fears and our emotional wounds.

So the shadow has two sides: dark and golden.

The dark shadow contains the rejected traits that we deem to be negative or harmful, such as anger, fear and shame, while our golden shadow is made up of our hidden talents, our blinding beauty and our unfulfilled potential – traits that we often also reject or keep hidden.

Just as the dark shadow is made up of all the parts of ourselves that we fear may lead to rejection, so the golden shadow is made up of all the bright, brilliant and magnificent parts of ourselves that we fear may be too great, too awesome or too challenging to reveal to ourselves and others.

We will explore how we can use lucid dreaming for shadow integration practically in Chapter 7, but fundamentally it can be used to face our fears or to embrace our golden potential with compassionate acceptance. Just as the inner child will often appear in personified or physicalized form in our lucid dreams, so will the shadow. Over the past 20 years, I've invoked and hugged (the greatest expression of integration in a lucid dream) literally dozens of dark shadow aspects in the form of mobsters, the devil and scenarios of doom, plus loads of golden shadow aspects in the form of spiritual teachers, balls of light and symbols of transformation.

This process of engaging shadow aspects with the aim of integrating and assimilating them into the Self is part of what Jung termed 'individuation' – the move towards psychological wholeness. This is one of the highest aims of psychological work, so we can see how lucid dreaming offers us an arena in which to reconnect with these deep levels of our psyche, so that when we wake in the morning, we may feel very different from the day before.

Charlie says

'If shadow integration sounds like your cup of tea, then check out my third book, Dreaming Through Darkness, *or its new iteration,* Do the Shadow Work, *which are dedicated to the topic and show you how to integrate your shadow in the waking state as well as in dreams.'*

Having Fun!

Our final benefit is just as important as the rest. If something is fun, we are much more likely to actually do it, and neurochemically, pleasure can be profoundly good for us. Lucid dreaming allows you to do everything you've ever dreamed of doing. Whatever fantasy you choose, it's there for you in the hyperrealistic dream world of lucid awareness. You can be a movie star, have mad sexual orgies, experience psychedelic states and enjoy whatever your inner hedonist could wish for.

When I first taught myself to lucid dream at the age of 16, I used my newly found hobby for nothing more than sex, drugs and skateboarding. I wasted the first two years of my lucid dreaming practice almost exclusively on having sex in lucid dreams. At the time this felt like nothing more than harmless fun, and in fact it acted as a great motivational tool for me to get lucid as much as possible, but alas, it became a slippery slope down which I fell many times. For, as the great Irish poet W.B. Yeats said, 'In dreams begins responsibility.'[14] In lucid dreams, even more so.

As in waking life, we are always creating and strengthening neural pathways while we are lucid dreaming, which means that if we engage in unbeneficial actions while lucid, we are creating neurological pathways associated with that action, which can then become activated in the waking state. Hence the slippery slope.

And if we consider the concept of karma (cause and effect), then once we're lucid, we have volition and conscious motivation – the two driving forces behind karmic imprints. This means karma is engaged in a similar way to when we are awake, so harmful acts in a lucid dream will leave negative karmic traces, just as they would in waking reality. So, have fun, but be careful what you get up to in the lucid dream state and try to treat it as a sacred space rather than a playground.

That said, lucid dreaming is incredible fun. Flying, for example, feels as real as it would in the waking state. Like to travel? Try your hand at teleportation. Become invisible. Visit the moon. The sky's the limit.

So far we've concentrated on the psychological benefits, and soon we'll move on to the spiritual ones, but before we do, let's explore the spiritual tradition from which so many of these benefits come: Tibetan Buddhism.

CHAPTER 4
SLEEPING BUDDHAS

*'What happened to the Buddha is
comparable, or is similar to, the experience
that each of us has every morning when
the alarm goes off and we wake up.'*

Stephen Batchelor[1]

About 2,500 years ago, five centuries before Jesus, a young
Sakyan prince in the foothills of the Himalayas became the
original rich-kid dropout. His name was Siddhartha Gautama. At
the age of 29, after a palatial life of luxury during which he had been
kept blissfully ignorant of the suffering of the world, he decided
to radically change both his lifestyle and his mind. He wanted to
wake up.

The moment we wake up from a dream, we gain a lucid
insight – what we have taken as real has actually been a dream, an
intricate illusion. This is what happened to the Buddha, the only
difference being that whereas we wake from dreams to waking
reality, he woke from waking reality to ultimate reality.

Buddhism: Teachings on How to Wake Up

I started formally practising Buddhism when I was 19 and even lived at a Tibetan Buddhist centre, Kagyu Samye Dzong, in London for seven years. Since then, I have received teachings from some of the leading meditation masters and most esteemed gurus on the planet. What knowledge do I have to show for it? Very little. What enlightened qualities do I now possess? None. So, what do I have to show for over two decades of mind training? I am much kinder and friendlier than I used to be.

Buddhism is all about kindness and friendliness: unconditional kindness towards ourselves and others, unconditional friendliness towards pain and happiness, joy and despair. For me, that's the essence of the Buddha's teachings – unconditional kindness and friendliness towards everything.

Buddha himself summed up his message as: 'Do no harm, be kind and tame your mind.' A true Buddhist practitioner tries to engage in as many forms of wise, loving, kind, compassionate action as possible, while avoiding actions that do harm to themselves or others.

Charlie says

'Being kind doesn't mean being a doormat. Being kind to yourself means setting strong boundaries, and sometimes the kindest thing you can do in a situation might actually be quite forceful. Some of the kindest things people have done for me have been to point out my mistakes. Being kind doesn't always mean being nice.'

In the words of one Buddhist teacher, 'If you wonder what Buddhism has to offer you, the answer is: nothing. If you think that becoming a Buddhist will bring you all sorts of goodies and fringe benefits, forget it. What it can help you do is cut through your confusion and your neuroses. Buddhism can help you understand yourself.'[2]

This practical self-understanding is a recurring theme throughout the teachings, as are compassion and wisdom. Compassion without wisdom becomes blind sentimentality, which can often do more harm than good, but when coupled with insightful wisdom, it can be applied in a way that really works. Wisdom is the cultivation of insight into how things really are and the Buddha taught that one of the best ways to cultivate this insight was through meditation.

Meditation is a system of relaxed reflection and mind training that leads to awareness and insight. Meditating and reflecting bring us into direct contact with what is happening with our inner environment, so that we come to know ourselves better. And the better we know ourselves, the better equipped we are to help others.

The Buddha didn't set out to found a religion or to convert people to a belief – he simply taught a system of ethics, compassion and loving-kindness towards all beings that aimed to help people wake up to their own enlightened nature. He said, 'Don't blindly believe what I say. Find out for yourself what is truth, what is real.'

His teaching tools were meditation techniques that tamed the selfish mind and practical guidelines on how to live joyfully with wisdom and compassion. These tools are as applicable today as they were 2,500 years ago; in fact, the more modern science discovers about the nature of the mind, the more the Buddha's teachings ring true. Eventually they became 'Buddhism' – both a religion and a way of life that has spread around the globe.

There are three main schools of Buddhism: Theravada (the teachings of the elders), Mahayana (the greater vehicle) and Vajrayana (the diamond vehicle). We will focus primarily on Vajrayana, which flourished first in Northern India and then later in Tibet and the Himalayan region and was developed with two unique aims in mind: enlightenment within one lifetime and 24-hour spiritual practice.

Dreaming on the Roof of the World

Dreams have played a central role in Buddhism ever since the 'conception dream' of the Buddha's mother, Maya. In fact, the notion of conscious dreaming was put forth by the Buddha himself. In the *Pali Vinaya*, the original rulebook for Buddhist monks and nuns, the Buddha actually instructs his followers to fall asleep in a state of mindfulness as a way of preventing 'seeing a bad dream' or 'waking unhappily'.[3] So it seems that the healing potential of mindful sleeping goes right back to the source.

However, the first fully integrated system of lucid dream work within Buddhism would only appear more than 1,000 years later, when Vajrayana found its way to Tibet. There it encountered an indigenous form of mysticism called Bön, which had a long history of shamanic dream practices.

Both of these traditions practised lucid dreaming, so it's not surprising that in Tibetan Buddhism in particular we find dreams playing such an important role.

Tibetan folklore and the biographies of Buddhist saints are littered with references to dreams. In Tibetan Buddhism itself, dreams are indispensably significant insofar as they are used to find reincarnated masters, to predict future events and to receive spiritual teachings. Recognition of their significance led to the development of a systematic path of practice called dream yoga.

Tibetan Dream Yoga

It would be easy to say that dream yoga was a Tibetan Buddhist form of lucid dreaming, but that would also be lazy and inaccurate. Dream yoga, *milam naljor* in Tibetan, is a collection of transformational lucid dreaming, conscious sleeping and what in the West we refer to as out-of-body-experience practices aimed at spiritual growth, mind training and full awakening. Lucid dreaming may form the foundation of dream yoga but, through the use of advanced tantric energy work, visualizations of Tibetan iconography and the integration of psycho-spiritual archetypes or *yidams*, dream yoga goes way beyond our Western notion of lucid dreaming.

The Sanskrit word *yoga* means 'union' and dream yoga is about the union of consciousness within the dream state. It is a yoga of the mind that uses advanced lucid dreaming methods to utilize sleep on the path to spiritual awakening.

Within Buddhism, illusion and ignorance* are seen as two of the most unbeneficial mind states and there are thousands of practices that aim to transmute them. One of these is dream yoga. Once we're fully lucid in a dream, ignorance is challenged as we recognize that what we thought was real is in fact not real. At the same time, illusion is shattered as we recognize that the entire dreamscape is formed from a mental projection.

As ignorance and illusion dissolve, two highly beneficial states of mind can arise in their place: insight and wisdom. Insight arises as we see clearly that we are dreaming, and wisdom dawns as we understand that our mind is creating our experience. Through dream yoga we can transmute ignorance and illusion while generating wisdom and insight, all while we're sound asleep.

In some lineages, dream yoga was reserved for those on a three-year retreat and was only taught as part of the famous Six Yogas of Naropa.** These days, however, some of the veils of secrecy have been lifted, allowing it to become a practice that enables dedicated practitioners to extend meditative awareness throughout sleep and dreams, and subsequently throughout death and dying as well.

---

* Within Buddhism, ignorance doesn't mean 'stupidity', it means 'not knowing what really is'. So, a non-lucid dream is a dream of ignorance because we think it's real and don't know that it's a dream.

** Naropa was a 10th-century *mahasiddha* who founded the Karma Kagyu school of Tibetan Buddhism. The Six Yogas of Naropa are a series of advanced tantric practices designed to bring the practitioner to full spiritual realization within one lifetime.

Dreams and death are closely linked in Tibetan Buddhism, as we will explore throughout this book.

The Dalai Lama has said, 'Dream yoga can be practised by both Buddhists and non-Buddhists alike',[4] and that through dream yoga the lucid dreamer can engage in spiritual practice while they sleep. So, I encourage you not to feel excluded from this esoteric-sounding practice if you're not a Buddhist. Although some of the advanced dream yoga techniques should only be engaged in under the guidance of a qualified teacher, there are many techniques that you can practise on your own. We will explore some of these in Part II. Ultimately, it's the motivation behind dream yoga that's the most important aspect of all, fuelling the use of lucid dreaming as a path to spiritual awakening.

Bardo: *The Place in Between*

Bardo is a Tibetan word that means 'place in between' and is used to describe any transitional state of existence. Just as dreaming is the *bardo* between falling asleep and waking up, life is the *bardo* between birth and death. However, what I want to focus on now is the after-death *bardo*, which describes the intermediate states between death and rebirth.

'Sleep', 'death' and 'dreams' all have the same root syllables in Sanskrit. In the Buddhist tradition, sleep isn't just a metaphor for death, as it is in the West, it is actually the prime training ground for death. Why? Because the after-death *bardo* state is said to be dreamlike in nature. So, it's believed that if we gain mastery over the mind of dreams then we will also have mastery over the mind of death. If we can fall asleep consciously and then recognize our dreams as dreams, we may also be able to die consciously and recognize the dreamlike after-death *bardo* state.

In his book *Living, Dreaming, Dying*, the recently deceased Buddhist teacher Rob Nairn says:

When we die, our stream of consciousness floats free from the body and roams the death bardos (the dreamlike hallucinatory experience that the mindstream enters into once it has separated from the physical body at the point of death). The mind is nine times stronger in this state and so if it is able to focus on spiritual truth, it will immediately be drawn into it, experience it and be liberated by it into awakening.[5]

He goes on to say:

In the death bardos our enlightened reality appears to us over and over again, and if the bardo mind can focus sufficiently to recognize the experience for what it is... the result will be immediate enlightenment.[6]

So, clearly, it is understood that if practitioners can become fully lucid within the death and after-death *bardo* states, they have the potential to recognize the nature of their mind and reach full spiritual awakening. Dream yoga is the core training for this potential.

Buddhist scholar B. Alan Wallace says that within Buddhism it is believed that 'among the three general states of consciousness – waking, sleeping and dreaming – the coarsest state of consciousness, the one with the least potential for spiritual development, is, surprisingly, the ordinary waking state'.[7] So, the dream and sleep states actually have more potential for spiritual development than daily life.

Tibetan Buddhism divides dreams into three main classes: ordinary samsaric dreams, dreams of clarity and clear light experiences.

Samsara is the term used to denote cyclic existence – the experience of birth, life, death and rebirth as perpetuated by dualistic ignorance. It is the antithesis of *nirvana*, enlightenment, and until we are enlightened, we are stuck in *samsara*. Psychologically, it could be thought of as 'going round in circles', the repetition of fruitless emotional patterns and reactive mental narratives sourced from a belief in a permanently existing self. Samsaric dreams reflect this and simply consist of all our non-lucid dreams about our mental preoccupations and memories from this life, and perhaps previous lives, too.

Dreams of clarity are decidedly different – they include what we in the West call lucid dreams and are considered very beneficial. They may range from witnessing dreams to high-level super-lucid dreams. They may also include dreams of significant insight (in which we may not necessarily be lucid), prophetic dreams and the kind of transpersonal dream experiences that Carl Jung called 'big dreams'.

Clear light experiences go a significant step further. They are experiences in which we discover the true nature of our own mind – beyond, and apart from, our deluded projections, and beyond subject–object duality. To try to describe clear light experiences in words is a struggle, but it's safe to say that they are not so much dreams as experiences of non-dual awareness accessed through sleep. We will touch on the Clear Light of Sleep in Chapter 8.

To understand the Tibetan Buddhists' perspective on dreaming, it helps to understand what they mean by wakefulness. Wakeful experience is perceived not quite as the solid reality we persistently assume it to be, but rather as a dreamlike illusion, a subjective projection based on the impermanent and interdependent nature of all phenomena. It's not quite as simple as saying, 'Everything is a dream,' but more as if waking reality is viewed as dreamlike in nature and not as 'real' as we tend to regard it. Of course on a relative, everyday level, things do exist – bills need to be paid and the laws of the universe apply – but on the level of enlightened understanding, waking life is not viewed as a fully awakened state, but as a dreamlike mirage through which we are sleepwalking. In other words, in Tibetan Buddhism, the dream that we experience during sleep is actually a dream within a dream, or a 'secondary illusion' to the 'primary illusion' of waking life.

In his book *Sleeping, Dreaming, and Dying*, the Dalai Lama comments, 'If you ask why we dream, what's the benefit, there is no answer in Buddhism'[8] – other than its use in meditative practice.

So it could be said that from the perspective of Tibetan Buddhism, the benefits of dreaming are only truly met by engaging in meditative sleep practices such as lucid dreaming. Once we recognize that we are dreaming, the dream state can become a potential workshop of enlightened action and spiritual growth in which mindful awareness, compassionate action and the dissolution of negative mental tendencies can transform our mind at the deepest level.

The practices of lucid dreaming and dream yoga are not only intended to train the practitioner to become lucid within the after-death *bardo*, but also to train them to become lucid in the waking state. This lucid awakening within the shared dream of life is exactly what transformed Siddhartha Gautama into the Buddha. This is an awakening that is possible for us all.

Now that we've seen how lucid dreaming and dream yoga sit within the ancient Vajrayana Buddhist tradition, let's explore some of the tangible benefits and see just how deep this practice can take us.

CHAPTER 5

THE SPIRITUAL BENEFITS OF LUCID DREAMING

'Most people have not yet fully understood the real potential of lucid dreaming. But once people know how important this is, everyone will practise it!'

Lama Yeshe Rinpoche[1]

The spiritual benefits we'll explore in this chapter are presented mainly from the perspective of Tibetan Buddhism because that's the spiritual tradition of which I am part, but these benefits aren't limited to Buddhists. Whatever your take on life and spirituality, lucid dreaming has so much to offer you.

Preparation for Death

Each day 150,000 people do it and one day we will do it, too. No matter where we're from or who we are, it is the one experience we will all share – the great equalizer. We will all do it and we will all do it successfully. We will all die. So, in the words of Buddhist master Dzogchen Ponlop Rinpoche,* we have a choice: 'to prepare

---

* *Rinpoche* means 'precious one' in Tibetan and is used as a term of reverence for high lamas and esteemed masters. It is pronounced with emphasis on the 'e' so that it rhymes with 'cabaret'.

ourselves to face the most uncomfortable moment of our lives or to meet that moment unprepared'.[2]

Most of us in the West sleep for about 30 years of our lives, but how long do we spend contemplating death – an hour, a day, a week? I propose we start redressing this imbalance and start waking up to the reality of our mortality. While we are alive we have a wonderful opportunity to prepare ourselves for death, so let's try to get over our defence mechanism of death denial and take some time to prepare.

One of the best preparations for death is through lucid dreaming and conscious sleeping. Within Tibetan Buddhism, as already mentioned, the main purpose of these sleep and dreaming practices is preparation for the dreamlike after-death *bardo* state. Each time we fall asleep and dream, we're getting a trial run for death and dying,* so every time we fall asleep consciously or have a lucid dream, we're training for the conscious recognition of the death process and the after-death *bardo*.

According to the *Tibetan Book of the Dead*, if we can manage to recognize the dreamlike hallucinations of the 49-day after-death *bardo* state as manifestations of the mind, we have the possibility of experiencing full spiritual awakening. It is said that even if a yogi has practised meditation for a whole lifetime and still hasn't attained full realization, he has one last shot at it: death. My teacher and dream yoga master, Lama Yeshe Rinpoche, once told me, 'If you want to know how your mind will be during death, look at how your mind is during a dream. If you can remember to recognize the dream consistently, then death means nothing to you, because you can recognize the death *bardo* as a dream, and then you can be with Buddha.'

---

* Within the Tibetan teachings, the process of falling asleep corresponds to the dissolution of the four elements (earth, water, fire and air) that occurs at death.

When it's 4 a.m. and my alarm has gone off, reminding me to write down my dreams and practise lucid dreaming, it's that quote that spurs me on. Sure, we can use our lucid dreams to do loads of cool stuff that will help us while we're alive, but some of the greatest benefits of this practice come when we die.

Spiritual Practice While We Sleep

The great Tibetan masters recommend that we use our lucid dreams to do our spiritual practice while we sleep. Within Tibetan Buddhism it is believed that 'the mind is up to seven times more powerful'[3] in the lucid dream state, meaning that any spiritual practice that we do is charged with up to seven times the power.

In fact, doing spiritual practice in the lucid dream state is said to be so powerful that we have the potential to reach full enlightenment while we sleep. The first Karmapa, the spiritual head of the Kagyu school of Tibetan Buddhism, attained full enlightenment at the age of 50 while practising dream yoga. So we shouldn't think that spiritual practice in the lucid dream state is somehow second best to waking practice – it can be even more effective.

In his book *Tibetan Dream Yoga: The Royal Road to Enlightenment*, Dr Michael Katz testifies to this when he says that 'there may be extraordinary results from intentionally doing spiritual practice within a lucid dream' and that 'one moment of spiritual practice in a lucid dream is equivalent to one week of spiritual practice in the waking state'.[4]

What exactly is meant by 'spiritual practice' here? It's simple. Once lucid within a dream, engage in Buddhist meditation or Christian prayer, shamanic visualization, Hindu mantra recitation or whatever spiritual practice you do in the same way you would in the waking state. This is not only a great way to spend our dreaming hours, it's also incredibly powerful, because our dream body is unhindered by the physical limitations of our waking body, meaning that we have the potential to reach levels of accomplishment that may seem impossible in the waking state. Energy work such as *tai chi* or *chi gong* depends in part upon the movement and flow of energy through our body, which in the waking state can often be disrupted by internal bodily blockages. In the lucid dream state, however, our dream body is pure energy with no physical form, which means that these types of energy practices can be engaged in to their maximum potential.

In Tibetan Buddhism, certain meditation practices require that we visualize ourselves taking on the actual form and qualities of a specific buddha, or archetype of enlightened energy. If we engage in this within a lucid dream, we can transform into the actual form of the buddha and experience an aspect of their luminous nature while we sleep.

The first time I tried this in a lucid dream, I visualized myself as the buddha of compassion, Chenrezig, who is symbolized as a buddha with snow-white skin and four arms. Soon I started to feel an incredible buzzing sensation throughout my entire dream body. I felt as if I was exuding power from every pore, but a power of pure love and kindness. I then felt my dream body transform into the form of Chenrezig! (*For a full description of this dream, see Dream 3, page 259, and for the instructions on how to do this specific practice, see page 123.*)

Psychologically, this kind of practice leaves an indelible imprint on our mindstream, and physiologically, 'research shows that the dream environment is even more effective for establishing neural connections'[5] than waking visualization. So, our lucid dreams can reveal our limitless potential for enlightened manifestation. And, crucially, this serves to supercharge our waking spiritual practice, too.

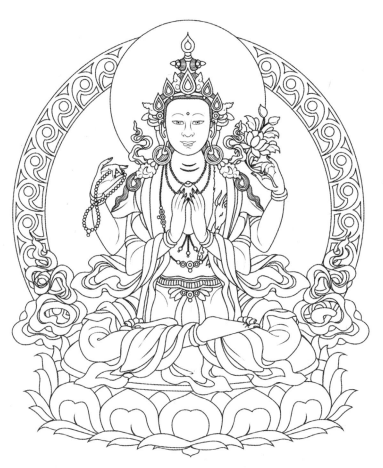

Chenrezig, the buddha of compassion

Exploring Emptiness

Shunyata, often translated as 'emptiness', is a Buddhist term used to describe the impermanent and interdependent nature of all phenomena. What it suggests is that reality is in fact a dreamlike illusion, empty of all inherent solid existence.

I've heard some teachers say that *shunyata* should actually be translated as 'pure potentiality' – things aren't empty because they are lacking something, but because they contain infinite potentiality. Whatever way you look at it, the concept of *shunyata* is admittedly quite far out, even for practising Buddhists. As one Tibetan lama says, 'Emptiness will freak you out! Good freak you out, but still freak you out!'[6]

It isn't just a concept, though – it has a practical application for our own happiness. As Dzigar Kongtrul Rinpoche says in his book *It's Up to You*:

> Seeing the emptiness of the world relieves us of the heavy notion of things being so solid. When we understand that nothing exists independently, everything that does arise seems more dreamlike and less threatening. Because the nature of everything is emptiness, we can relax and enjoy the show.[7]

In a lucid dream we know that however solid, real and separate things may seem, they are actually illusions created by our own mind. So, through lucid dreaming we directly experience a facet of emptiness. It is said that 'through dream yoga the yogi can directly recognize the emptiness of the personal self and of phenomena',[8] because if we can experience how convincingly real things are in our lucid dreams, we may become better able to experience the dreamlike nature of waking reality, too.

Through lucid dreaming we learn to combat grasping at the seemingly solid reality of waking existence, because we know what it feels iike to be conscious within a similarly 'real' dream state that we know is in fact an absolute figment of our imagination.

Seeing through the illusion of dualistic reality is all part of the process of spiritual awakening, but it is an experience that can be hard to muster in a world that seems so solid and separate from ourselves. A lucid dream offers us a rare training ground for this experience, because, as my teacher Rob Nairn once said, through lucid dreaming 'we experience the realization that what we thought to be real is actually not real, and so we are no longer experiencing the ignorance of the illusion. This is a taste of awakening.'[9]

Charlie says

'If all this emptiness stuff seems a bit far out, it's worth noting that quantum physics supports the idea, in principle at least, because 99.9999999999999 per cent of an atom is empty space, meaning that if we were to force together all the atoms of all the humans who had ever lived and then to remove the empty space in those atoms, the entire human race would fit into an area the size of a sugar cube.[10] Now that really is far out.'

Receiving Teachings

Every one of us has an aspect of innate wisdom, often called the 'higher self', 'enlightened potential' or 'Buddha nature', which is always within us. In the waking state this inner wisdom can often seem quite elusive, but in a lucid dream it is much easier to access, because the layers of ignorance that obscure our naturally enlightened mind are less dense.

While we are lucid, this inner wisdom will often offer us teachings spontaneously, taking on the form of an archetype of wisdom from our personal belief system – Jesus for one person, white light for another. Although the teachings may seem to come from a separate entity, they are, for the most part, sourced from within ourselves, from a potential that many of us are unaware we possess.

Having said that, we might also be able to receive teachings from the subtle energy mindstreams of enlightened beings. It seems to be far easier to tune into these mindstreams from the lucid dream state than from the waking state. Lama Tsongkhapa, the teacher of the first Dalai Lama, taught that one of the core aims of dream yoga was to receive teachings within the lucid dream from buddhas, enlightened masters and spiritual guides. Within this tradition, we are encouraged to request teachings from these enlightened sources once we are in a lucid dream.

In the Celtic tradition, seers spoke of 'thin places' – leyline intersections or underground springs or other special sites where the boundary between the mundane and mystical was 'thin' and permeable. I believe that the lucid dream state is a similarly 'thin' place, with boundaries that are partially permeable, allowing us to access not only our own inner wisdom with greater ease, but also the enlightened energy of other beings.

On many occasions I've called out for and received direct teachings within my lucid dreams from beings that appeared to be separate entities who had entered my dream state. Due to the interconnected nature of all things, of course these entities were as much projections of my own enlightened potential as they were seemingly separate from me.

But however they are delivered, are the teachings we receive in lucid dreams to be taken seriously? I believe that if they encourage us to be kinder and more compassionate to ourselves and others, then we should put them into action – and only then. That's the safest option.

According to the great dream yogi Norbu Rinpoche, if we are truly aware in the dream state, a teaching received within the dream 'has the same value'[11] as a teaching received in the waking state, but he advises that we should apply discernment to all teachings, dream or waking, rather than accepting them out of blind faith.

Lucid Living

I have a friend named Tim Freke. He often says, 'With a name like mine, I guess I had to become a philosopher.' And so he did. One of Tim's areas of expertise is Christian Gnosticism and the concept of lucid living that the Gnostics proposed. Waking up to life and living lucidly was a central concept for these mystic proto-Christians, as we can see from their call to 'Wake up! Rouse yourself from the collective coma that you mistake for "real life"!'[12]

The Gnostics believed that we were sleepwalking through the illusion of waking reality, unaware that it was all just as empty of inherent existence as our dreams. If only we could get lucid in our waking reality, maybe we would see that life was but a dream?

Far from trying to wake up, most of us willingly surrender 30 years of our life to non-awareness. Each night we fall into an abyss of ignorance, surrendering seven to nine hours to unconsciousness, and then wake up in the morning as if this is the most natural thing in the world. We are in fact conditioned to see it as normal and to view sleep as a time of complete non-awareness, a time to 'switch off the computer', but it doesn't have to be this way.* Although much of sleep *is* about the body and brain shutting down, the time spent in dreaming sleep is not, and so, as the dream yogi Tenzin Wangyal Rinpoche says, 'These dream practices can help us not to waste that time but to spend it learning to discover our inner potential. What a fantastic tool!'[13]

When we learn that we may be losing 30 years to total lack of awareness, our rational mind might counter with 'Yeah, maybe, but at least I'm wide awake and living lucidly for the rest of it!' Unfortunately, this simply isn't true. Studies from a Harvard University research team have found that most people are unaware

---

* Much of sleep is about restoration, but we don't have to be unconscious for this restoration to occur. Conscious sleeping and lucid dreaming practices will make our sleep *more* refreshing, not less so.

and not in the present moment for 47 per cent of their waking lives.[14] The researchers concluded that most of us live our lives on autopilot, lost in fantasy and very rarely present and mindful. Most of us are definitely not living lucidly, but every time we have a lucid dream we are habituating our mind to be more aware and lucid in our waking lives, too.

In a lucid dream, we become aware that what we believed to be real (the dream) is not real but just a mental projection. By becoming lucid, we see through our projections, and each time we do that, we are creating a habitual tendency towards seeing through our projections in the waking state, too.

Projection describes a psychological defence mechanism in which we unconsciously project our own unacceptable qualities onto others. For example, if we are arrogant, we may deny this in ourselves but see it in others to a degree not quite proportionate to reality. The arrogance of others becomes exaggerated in our eyes and 'pushes our buttons'. In fact, what annoys us most in other people is often a trait we are working hard not to recognize and accept in ourselves. Projection runs rife.

Once we establish a stabilized lucid dreaming practice, however, we stabilize a new power of recognition that can 'see through' projections, not only of the dream type, but of the waking type too. This is how we begin to live lucidly, because we start to recognize our waking psychological projections in the same way as we recognize our dreams.

Through learning to dream lucidly, we can learn to live lucidly and wake up to life. Perhaps we can even realize what those early Gnostic Christians were getting at when they said, 'You are asleep and dreaming. Wake up. How can you bear to be asleep when it's your responsibility to be awake?'[15]

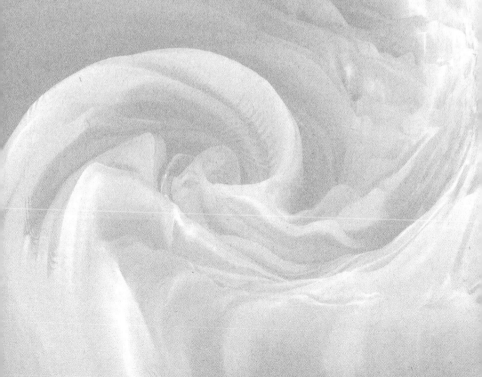

PART II

PATH

CHAPTER 6

DAYTIME LUCID DREAMING TECHNIQUES

'Where are you right now?'

'Oh my God. We're dreaming?'

'You're actually in the middle of the workshop right now, sleeping. This is your first lesson... Stay calm.'

Inception, directed by Christopher Nolan

Now that we've prepared the ground, answered some of the most frequently asked questions and have a broad outline of the history and benefits of the practice, it's time to move on to the actual path of lucid dreaming. This part of the book will give you a toolbox of techniques with which you can learn to dream lucidly.

In the ancient Buddhist dream yoga teachings, the techniques are often separated into daytime techniques and night-time techniques. Although we aren't quite following exactly the same classification, I have divided the practices into ones that you do while awake and ones that you do while falling asleep or dreaming.

> **Charlie says**
>
> 'With so much of lucid dream induction being dependent upon intention, our actual preparation for sleep can be used as a lucid dreaming technique in itself. Set and setting are key. If we take some time before sleep to prepare the space of both our sleeping area and our mind, we will imbue our final minutes of wakefulness with the strong intention for lucidity.'

All the practices that we will explore here are taken from both Western and Tibetan Buddhist sources. Although some Tibetan dream yoga techniques can't be shared outside a formal retreat setting, don't feel that you're missing out on the complete package, because, as one high lama says, 'Training in dream yoga is similar to the methods developed by Western researchers. Both the Western exercises and the Tibetan methods can be used, since they are essentially the same thing.'[1]

The following practices show us how to wake up to the dream of life as well as the dream of the night and help us to train in lucid living as well as lucid dreaming. These techniques can be practised by people of all faiths and levels of ability, and each one has been tested, refined and successfully applied by the thousands of dreamers that I've taught at retreats, workshops and lectures in more than 25 countries around the world.

I've seen the following practices transform people's lives. So let's start!

What's Your Motivation?

Getting lucid won't happen just by reading about lucid dreaming – it's all about *practising* lucid dreaming. Just as looking at a map won't get you anywhere, reading this book won't give you lucid dreams – you need to set out on the path.

Dr Stephen LaBerge famously said that there are three essential requirements for learning to lucid dream: excellent *dream recall*, correct practice of *effective techniques* and *strong motivation*. The dream recall and effective techniques can be taught, but the motivation is down to each one of us individually.

So, is your motivation just to have a bit of fun or to try to make use of your sleep for psychological growth? Either option is fine, but there's a third option too: to use these practices to wake up to your highest potential.

The Tibetan Buddhist masters say that we should try to imbue our dream practice with '*bodhicitta** motivation', which means that we are motivated to have lucid dreams not just for our own benefit, but to awaken our deeper capacity for wisdom and compassion, which will benefit other beings too. That seems a pretty sensible motivation, whether you're a Buddhist or not, but how can lucid dreaming be used to benefit others? It's said that every time you get lucid, wisdom is accumulated, because you are gaining insight into illusion and increasing your capacity for mindful awareness, which is the bedrock of love and compassion. Essentially, by becoming lucid in our dreams, we become more lucid, insightful and compassionate in our waking lives – and that can only be of benefit to both others and ourselves.

Charlie says

'*Lucid dreaming makes us kinder in everyday life. It shows us how our mind creates illusion, which allows us to see how other people's minds do the same. Once we see that, we realize that everybody is trying their best and that we're all in this together. We become a bit more tolerant and responsive, rather than closed and reactive.*'

---

* *Bodhicitta* is one of the most important aspects of Tibetan Buddhism. It's the wish to attain enlightenment not just for ourselves, but for the benefit of all beings (Sanskrit: *bodhi* = enlightened essence; *citta* = heart/mind).

The Four 'D's

One of the big changes that has occurred since the first edition of this book was published in 2013 is how much media attention lucid dreaming has had. I've done literally hundreds of podcasts, press interviews and TV slots over the past 10 years, and invariably one of the last questions I am asked is: 'So, how do we actually do it?' and I then have the seemingly impossible task of trying to teach lucid dreaming in five minutes or less!

Over the years, though, I've developed a pretty good way of doing so that I call the four 'D's:

1. Dream Planning

2. Dream Recall

3. Dream Diary

4. Dream Signs

Here's a brief explanation that not only lays out the road map for the first few techniques we'll explore but also gives you a good five-minute elevator pitch, should anyone ask you how they can start their own lucid dream training.

Dream Planning

First of all, decide what you want to do in your first or next lucid dream by creating a dream plan. What do you plan to do in your lucid dreams and why? Which one of the benefits that we've just learned about do you want to explore?

Having a good reason *why* is the most powerful lucid dream induction technique there is.

Dream Recall

The second 'D' is dream recall. Recalling your dreams is essential to lucid dreaming, because 'the more conscious you are of your dreams, the easier it will be to become conscious within your dreams'.[2]

And you do definitely dream. Everyone does, every single night. In fact, it is impossible to stop the human brain from dreaming other than by having a stroke or a severe head injury, and even then dreaming will return within a few weeks.

So, you do dream, but maybe you don't remember your dreams? Here's how you can remedy this: simply set an intention to remember your dreams before you fall asleep. It sounds too simple to be true, but it really works.

As you fall asleep, keep telling yourself over and over, 'Tonight I remember my dreams. I have excellent dream recall.'

When you fall asleep, you pass through a state of consciousness called the hypnagogic state, which is a natural state of hypnosis, so this technique is essentially hypnotizing yourself to remember your dreams, and it usually works very well.

Once you have started remembering your dreams, the next step is to document them in some way. This is our third 'D': the dream diary.

Dream Diary

This is basically about writing down your dreams or documenting them in some way. How does that lead to lucidity exactly? It allows you to recognize the memory of an unconscious process (your dreams) with your conscious awareness. Through keeping a dream diary you are starting to make that link between conscious and unconscious.

And crucially, by writing down your dreams, you're mapping out the territory of your dreaming mind. The better you get to know that territory, the more likely you are to recognize it when you're actually in it and become lucid. Even if you can only remember a few flashes of your dreams, write them down – something is better than nothing.

As you write, you might start to recognize that the territory of your dreams often contains zombies or school scenes, so you are starting to make a link between the landmarks of your dreams and the fact that they only appear in your dreams. This is the crux of our fourth 'D': dream signs.

Dream Signs

A dream sign is any improbable, impossible or bizarre aspect of a dream experience that can indicate that you're dreaming. Often dreams are full of dream signs, which can be as subtle as being back at school and as obvious as flying pink elephants. Basically, if it's something that doesn't usually occur in waking life, then it's a potential dream sign.

Once you've pinpointed your dream signs, make a determined effort to be on the lookout for any future ones in subsequent dreams. This determined effort will carry over into your dreams and eventually you'll start recognizing dream signs from *within* the dream and become lucid.

And if you find that you have a recurring dream sign, such as your dead grandma, for example, try to use it as a lucidity trigger by saying repeatedly to yourself before bed, 'The next time I see my dead grandma, I'll know that I'm dreaming.' Then, when you next dream about your dead grandma, the lucidity trigger will be activated, making you spontaneously think, *Aha! This is a dream sign. I must be dreaming!*

•••

And now, because we have more than five minutes of a podcast together, let's explore each of the four 'D's in more depth.

Dream Planning

In the first edition of this book, dream planning only got a brief mention. Now it gets prime position, and is in my view the most important lucid dream induction technique of all, because if you have a good reason to lucid dream you'll have lucid dreams much, much more easily.

I advise you to 'go big' with your dream plan. Heal your wounded inner child, meet God, transform into a buddha, really shoot for the stars, and if it's too audacious or something that you're actually not ready for, know that your Dreamer, that intelligence of the dream state, will either dial it down for you or simply won't comply.

I teach dream planning in three main steps:

1. Writing a dream plan.

2. Drawing a dream plan (the dreaming mind works in images, so this helps).

3. Creating a *sankalpa* (a Sanskrit term meaning 'will' or 'purpose'), or statement of intent.

. . . .

Let's Make a Dream Plan!

First of all, draft some ideas of what you'd like to do in your first or next lucid dream. What would you do if you could do anything? What trauma would you like to integrate? What part of your shadow would you like to interact with? What spiritual practice would you like to do? What question would you like to ask your higher self?

Have a look over my recommended Top 10 dream plans (*pages 99–126*) for inspiration.

Once you've decided what you want to do, begin to formulate your dream plan.

Writing a dream plan

Using a fresh piece of paper, write at the top, 'In my next lucid dream I...' and then write a description of what you want to do once you become lucid. Focus less on the setting of the dream (you might become lucid in a totally random dreamscape) and more on what you want to do once you become lucid.

For example, 'In my next lucid dream I call out for my inner child. They appear in personified form and I embrace them with love. This embrace heals and integrates any and all wounded or traumatized aspects of my inner child and I wake up feeling transformed and totally healed.'

Charlie says

'Writing a dream plan is like writing a love letter to your dreaming mind, so don't be scared to ask for the most perfect, amazing lucid dream. It may not turn out exactly as you planned, but if you don't ask, you don't get, so write exactly what you would like to happen.'

Drawing a dream plan

Next, draw a picture of your dream plan in action. I just use stick men and speech bubbles, but if you're artistic, then of course feel free to do more. Your picture can be literal or abstract, simple or complex. Be creative – there are no rules for this.

Creating a *sankalpa*

Now write your *sankalpa*, or statement of intent. This should be a pithy statement that sums up the essence of your dream plan. It is your 'call to action'. For example, if my dream plan is a complex description of how I want to meet the personification of my relationship anxiety and embrace them with loving-kindness, my *sankalpa* might be: 'Heartbroken Charlie, come to me!'

Your dream plan description can be as long and detailed as you like, but I recommend that you keep your *sankalpa* short and sharp.

Before you go to bed, commit the *sankalpa* to memory, remind yourself of your dream plan and engage your favourite night-time lucid dream induction method (see *pages 127–156*).

The final step occurs when you next find yourself in a lucid dream. Once you get lucid, recall your dream plan, engage your *sankalpa* by either doing what you intended to do (meditating, for example) or by saying the *sankalpa* out loud* if it was an invocation or question.

And finally, engage in your chosen lucid activity with full confidence, holding in mind at all times the fact that you are dreaming.

. . . .

It may sound simplistic, but when you're operating in a world of mental constructs, it's your thoughts, words and expectations that dictate what happens, so really try to have full confidence that your dream plan will manifest as you want it to.

Charlie says

'Don't be too rigidly attached to your dream plan, though. If you plan to practise your surfing, but once you're lucid, the Dalai Lama appears and wants to give you the meaning of life, obviously just forget the surfing dream plan and go and hang out with the Dalai Lama!'

Here is an example of a full dream plan:

---

* Stating your intent mentally is fine, of course, but I recommend that beginners state their intent out loud, because that seems to help concretize it in a clearer and more precise way.

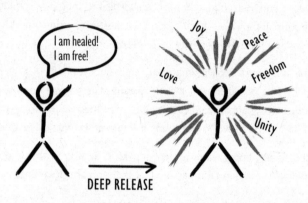

In my next lucid dream I will... heal the wounded part of myself by calling out within the dream: 'I am healed! I am free of my wounds! Wounded self, I love you!' As this happens, I experience a deeply beneficial integration of my psychological wounds and wake up feeling peaceful and healed.

> I am healed!
> I am free!

Joy

Peace

Love

Freedom

Unity

DEEP RELEASE

Sankalpa: 'I am healed! I am free of my wounds! Wounded self, I release you!'

A Threefold Manifestation

Creating a dream plan is a bit like creating a vision board or a manifestation anchor, so it can often have quite a strong effect on your life even before you have the lucid dream and carry it out.

Some people find that they have a non-lucid dream about their dream plan, as if their subconscious is so enthusiastic to engage it that it won't wait for the conscious mind to become lucid. If your dream plan is to heal the wounded inner child, for example, you may find that you have a non-lucid dream in which you are a child feeling happy and carefree – maybe not exactly what you had scripted in your dream plan, but a not dissimilar experience.

Others find that their dream plan manifests in the shared dream of waking reality, whereby the question that was posed in the dream plan is answered through some strange synchronicity or the healing that they wanted to do in the lucid dream spontaneously manifests in the waking state. This is not nearly as common, but I have seen it happen.

For most, though, the plan will manifest as intended, through a lucid dream. And once it's complete, create a new one.

Dream Recall

Now let's explore the bedrock of all dream work practices: recalling your dreams.

It took me years to appreciate fully just how vital dream recall is to lucidity. Initially, I thought it was just a way of making sure you remembered your dreams and a stepping stone to more advanced techniques. This isn't the case, though. Training in dream recall is essential, whatever your position on the path.

As mentioned earlier, recalling your dreams is essential to lucid dreaming because the more conscious you are of your dreams, the easier it will be to become conscious within your dreams.

Everybody dreams every night,[3] so why don't most people remember their dreams? There are all sorts of theories on this, ranging from it being maladaptive for early humans to remember their dreams (in case they confused them with reality) to ineffective modern sleeping patterns to a disregard for dreams in general, but I believe the reason people don't normally remember their dreams is simply because they don't *try* to remember them.

Dream recall is like ploughing the field of our unconscious, preparing it for the seeds of the lucidity techniques. We could just chuck a few seeds onto the field and a few might sprout, but if we plough the field properly, we'll get a much bigger harvest.

Dream recall is a great memory practice, too. It trains the mind to remember what it was up to while we were asleep and because it encourages us to flex our mindful memory muscles as soon as we wake up, it's great for our all-round mental health. If we set a strong intention to recall our dreams, most of us will be able to recall them without too much difficulty after just a couple of nights. It's all about intent.

Here are a few ways to boost your recall:

- Many people try to recall their dreams only after they have happened, but it's much better to set your intention to recall your dreams before you start dreaming. As you fall asleep, drifting through the hypnagogic state, keep reciting: 'Tonight I remember my dreams. I have excellent dream recall.' This simple method can be a profoundly effective remedy for dream amnesia.

- Knowing the time of your REM periods can be a great way to increase your recall, because if you wake people directly from REM sleep, most of them will be dreaming and will be able to describe what they were dreaming about. So, if you want to remember your dreams, try waking yourself during a REM period. REM periods get longer and occur at shorter intervals as the night progresses, so set an alarm clock for some time during the last two hours of your sleep cycle to have the best chance of waking up with dream recall. (*For more information, see 'The Stages of Sleep', page 128.*)

- Dream memories often seem to be stored in the muscle memory of our physical body, so for optimal dream recall, try not to move from the position in which you wake up until you can recall a dream. If you do have to move your body (to press the alarm clock, for example), return to the position in which you woke up and focus on recalling your dreams from there.

- Don't give up if you can't remember a dream straightaway. Often, my dreams come back to me while I'm having a cup of tea over breakfast, or sometimes even as late as the following afternoon when I become drowsy and my mind edges back to the dream state. Give yourself space to remember.

- Dream yogis say, 'Like a ball of yarn, even if we can only get the very end of the thread, we can work backwards and eventually unravel the entire dream.' So, even if you can only recall one fact or theme of the dream, you can work backwards from that point, eventually gathering the rest of it. As soon as you wake up, ask yourself: 'Where was I? What was I just doing? How am I feeling right now?'

- You can improve your dream recall by improving your waking recall, so train your memory muscles by asking yourself every few hours of the day, 'How did I get here?' and trace back your movements to the start of the day.

- The most important dream recall technique of all, though, is the first one we mentioned. As you're falling asleep, passing through the hypnotically suggestible hypnagogic state, recite over and over in your mind for at least a few minutes (or use your fingers to count 21 recitations if you want to follow the traditional Tibetan way): 'Tonight I remember my dreams. I have excellent dream recall.' This simple self-hypnosis method can be a profoundly effective remedy for people with dream amnesia. If they do this, most can recall at least part of their dreams without too much difficulty on the first or second night of trying.

Some people remember their dreams naturally, but for others it may take several days or even weeks of mental effort to do so. Whatever the state of your current dream recall, work with what you have and progress from there. Even if you can only recall a few fragments from each dream, that's a great start.

Dream Diary

Once you've set the strong intention to recall your dreams, the next step is to document them in some way.

Keeping a dream diary is simple: whenever you wake from a dream, recall as much of it as you can and write it down. You don't need to document every tiny detail; you'll know what's worth noting and what isn't. Five or ten minutes is all you need. Focus on the main themes and feelings, the general narrative and any strange anomalies that you can recall.

The idea is to get to know the territory of your dreams, the feel of your dreams and the shape of your dreams – three aspects that will help you to recognize your dreams when you are dreaming.

Nowadays many people make a note of their dreams on their phone (turn the screen brightness down, though), while others prefer pen and paper. If you're going to write up your dreams by hand, buy a notebook with paper that is a pleasure to write on, and use a pen that writes easily – do everything you can to encourage yourself to use your dream diary regularly.

Be sure to record the date of each dream at the top of the page* and feel free to give each dream a title – one that encapsulates it.

The Benefits of Keeping a Dream Diary

* Remember, it comes down to this: *The more conscious you are of your dreams, the easier it will be to become conscious within your dreams.*

---

* The importance of the date is so that once you start to have lucid dreams, you can chart your progress, and even cross-reference your dream diary with your everyday diary to see how your daily life influences your dreams.

- Writing down your dreams pays homage to the dreams and, more importantly, reinforces the habit of viewing them as something valuable. Once you see dreams as valuable, you will naturally start to recall them with more ease, and your dreaming mind may even respond by giving you dreams of more psychological value.

- Through the act of actually writing down your dreams you are recognizing the memory of an unconscious process with your conscious awareness. This will make your dreams manifest in a more conscious and recognizable way. *Recognizable* is the key word here, because the point of all these practices is to recognize that you're dreaming while you're dreaming.

- By writing down your dreams, you're mapping out the territory of your dreaming mind. The better you know that territory, the more likely you are to recognize it when you're in it and become lucid.

Top Tips for Keeping a Dream Diary

- Write down your dreams as soon as you remember them. Don't wait until the morning – do it straightaway. Countless times I've heard people say that they woke up in the night and recalled a dream so strongly that they were sure that they would still remember it in the morning, but in the morning it was gone!

- It can seem pretty hectic to scrabble around for your dream diary at 5 a.m., but you'll soon find the least disruptive method for you. Whether it's going to the bathroom to write up your dreams or having a little torch by your bedside to avoid waking your partner, you'll find a way.

- Many people, including myself, prefer making a note of their dreams on their phone (with the screen brightness turned down) and then printing them out at the end of each month.*

- Mind maps, illustrations, spider diagrams and artwork can all be incorporated into your dream diary. The important thing is to document your dreams in some way.

- Even if you can only remember a few fragments of a dream, write those down, and if you really can't remember anything, make a note of that, too.

- Voice recorders should be avoided if possible, though, because although it's difficult to 'sleep write', we can 'sleep talk'. If you try to record a dream into a voice recorder and you're not fully awake, you may well end up with a recording of yourself falling asleep!**

Charlie says

'Apart from leading to lucid dreams, keeping a dream diary gives you a nightly insight into the state of your mind. If you really want to know your own psychology, look at your dreams. They're an uncensored snapshot of you at that moment of your life. A dream diary is far more honest than a daytime diary, because your dreams don't lie nearly as much.'

---

* Whether you can afford half an hour documenting your dreams each morning or only five or ten minutes, either option is fine, but make sure you write something.

** In his book 59 Seconds Professor Richard Wiseman says, 'Talking can often be more unstructured, disorganized and by its nature improvised, in contrast to writing, which is more systematic and organized around structure.'[4]

Dream Signs

Once you've begun to recall your dreams, you can move on to spotting dream signs. A dream sign is any improbable, impossible or bizarre aspect of dream experience that can indicate that you're dreaming. Often dreams are full of dream signs, which can be as subtle as being in an unknown place and as obvious as talking to animals. Anything that doesn't usually occur in waking life is a potential dream sign.

There are hundreds of different types of dream signs, but I classify them into three main groups:

- *anomalous:* random one-off anomalies such as walking trees or barking cats

- *thematic:* themes or scenarios such as being back at school or naked in public

- *recurring:* dream signs that have appeared in two dreams or more on a weekly or monthly basis

By keeping a dream diary, we can log and record our particular dream signs and make notes of any recurring ones. Acknowledging our particular dream signs in the waking state will strengthen and cultivate what I call the 'critical reflective attitude of mind', and it is this cultivation that leads to the recognition of signs within the dream state, thus triggering lucidity.

Let's Spot Dream Signs!

Once you've recalled and written down your dreams, read back through them, on the lookout for dream signs. If you dreamed that you were walking down a street and saw former president Barack Obama standing next to a blue dragon, for example, then your dream signs would be 'Barack Obama' and 'blue dragon'. Unless you were Michelle Obama, of course, in which case seeing Barack Obama wouldn't be a dream sign, because he would be a feature of your everyday life. The blue dragon, however, would still be a dream sign. If you'd dreamed of a blue dragon several times, it would be a recurring dream sign. Recurring dream signs mean recurring opportunities to become lucid!

Once you've pinpointed your dream signs, set a strong intention to recognize them the next time they show up in your dreams, along with any future anomalies that might indicate that you're dreaming. This determined effort will seep into your dreams and eventually you'll start recognizing dream signs from within the dream.

If you spot a recurring dream sign, firmly resolve to use it as a lucidity trigger by saying to yourself over and over before bed: 'The next time I see a blue dragon, I'll know that I'm dreaming!' Then, when you next dream about your dream sign, the lucidity trigger will be activated, making you spontaneously think, *Blue dragon? Aha! This is a dream sign – I must be dreaming!* And you'll become lucid.

People often say, 'I've been having crazy dreams full of dream signs for years and I haven't been getting lucid!' This may well be because although their dreams have been full of dream signs, they haven't been acknowledging and labelling them as dream signs each morning. It is this process that strengthens the critical reflective attitude that leads to lucidity.

Charlie says

'It's so important to stress that simply by recognizing and acknowledging any dream sign, we strengthen the critical reflective habit of mind, a way of looking at our dreams in a more discerning way that is the driving force of lucidity.'

The most common way to enter into a lucid dream is simply to spot a dream sign and become lucid. This is what is called a DILD or Dream Initiated Lucid Dream. But sometimes, even though you've spotted a dream sign and are sure that you must be dreaming, the rest of the dream will look so realistic that you simply can't accept that you're in a dream. This is when you need a reality check.

Reality Checks

> *'You must start by doing something very simple. Tonight in your dreams you must look at your hands.'*
> **Don Juan, Yaqui Indian dream master[5]**

This is where it all gets a bit strange. Stephen LaBerge's Lucidity Institute has scientifically verified that there are certain things that are virtually impossible for the human mind to consistently replicate within the pre-lucid dream state* and so these can be used to reliably confirm whether or not you're dreaming. There are loads of them, but here are some of my favourites:

- looking at your outstretched hand twice in quick succession without it changing in some way

- reading text coherently twice without it changing in some way

- using digital or electrical devices without them changing or malfunctioning in some way

When I first read about these reality checks, I thought they were a load of BS (perhaps as you do now?), but try to stay with me on this, because once you know how they work, it all makes sense.

---

* Reality checks will almost always be performed in the pre-lucid dream state, because if you are conscious enough to think *I should do a reality check*, then you are often already pre-lucid.

During a dream, our brain is working flat out to maintain the projection of our elaborately detailed dreamscape in real time, and although it's amazingly good at this, once pre-lucid, it struggles to replicate the detailed minutiae of an intricate image such as a piece of text or an outstretched hand twice in quick succession. So, if we try to make it engage in such a replication, it will provide a close but imperfect rendering, and it's the acknowledgement of this imperfect rendering that makes us lucid.

Let's Check Reality!

Looking at your hand

You're in a dream and you see your dead grandma. You think you might be dreaming, but you're not 100 per cent sure; you're pre-lucid but not fully lucid. What to do? Look at your outstretched hand, then quickly look away and look back at it again. Alternatively, watch your hand as you flip it over and back again.*

Either way, your dreaming mind will try its best to reproduce exactly the same image, but won't quite have the processing speed to do so perfectly, so on second glance your hand may be a strange shape, perhaps missing a finger or two, or look dappled or transformed. I've seen my hand turn into a baby elephant and grow three new fingers!

The variations are multiple,** but the result is singular: something will change, and when it does, you'll know that you're definitely dreaming.

---

* This is one of the most applicable reality checks, because most people are embodied in their dreams and so a hand is always within reach.

** When Carlos Castaneda presses his teacher, Don Juan, about why he should look at his hands in particular, Don Juan replies, 'You can of course look at whatever you goddam please – your toes, your belly or even your pecker!'[6]

Charlie says

'I've had my hand turn into a tree, a robotic claw, a balloon and even just a stump of flesh. The dreaming mind is very creative, but it's not very good at replicating precise detail. Hands are pretty detailed, so it really struggles to replicate them to order.'

Reading text

Within a pre-lucid dream it is virtually impossible to read any text coherently twice in succession. LaBerge's research laboratory found that in lucid dreams text changed 75 per cent of the time as the dreamer was reading it and 95 per cent of the time on second reading.[7] So, if you're in a dream, see a dream sign and think you might be dreaming, try to read something. The text will often be unintelligible, move around as you're reading it or in some cases just fade away altogether. All these are signs that you're dreaming.*

Using digital and electrical appliances

Just as the dreaming mind struggles to reproduce text, it also struggles with the highly detailed screen of a mobile phone or computer, which will often seem blurred and fluid in a pre-lucid dream. I know it sounds crazy, but in a pre-lucid dream it's often virtually impossible to read a digital watch, successfully operate any form of digital or electrical appliance or switch a light on and off. This works on the principle that if you flick a light switch within a dream, you're asking the dreaming mind to project an exact replication of the dreamscape but in a totally different light and shadow setting, literally at the flick of a switch. This is something that it finds almost impossible.

---

* Perhaps this can be explained in part by the well-documented phenomenon whereby people recognize most words by their shape and so it *deosn't mttaer waht oredr ltteers appaer, olny taht the frist and lsat ltteers are in the rghit pclae.*

Until you've actually done a reality check, it can seem quite far-fetched, but let neuroscience put your mind at ease. Dreaming is mainly a right-brain activity, but when it comes to detailed information-processing, such as fluent reading, recognition of complex symbols and identifying detailed patterns, we rely almost solely on the superior processing speed of our left brain.[8] As this is much less active while we dream, if we try to process detailed information then, we'll be stumped. Working on this basis, we can see why all the reality checks that involve fluent reading and recreating detailed patterns are especially difficult within the dream state.

Interestingly, research has shown that once we actually have the 'Aha!' moment of lucidity, left-hemisphere function comes back online in about 30 seconds,[9] meaning that reality checks may become less necessary as the lucid dream progresses.

Charlie says

'Just to clarify, you don't have to do a reality check to become lucid; in fact, most lucid dreams are induced by simply recognizing a dream sign. Sometimes, though, you might recognize a dream sign but still not become fully lucid. In that situation you need a reality check.'

Although opportunities for reality checks will often crop up naturally in your dreams, they are usually only engaged once you spot a dream sign and need confirmation of your present reality. You can, however, actively hasten the process by getting into the habit of conducting reality checks while you're awake. This habit will naturally carry over into your dreams, so that soon you'll actually *dream* about doing a reality check, and if you do, it will reveal that you're dreaming. This is the basis of the Weird Technique...

The Weird Technique

This technique is deceptively simple, but it's how I used to have the majority of my lucid dreams. From now on, in the daytime, whenever something weird happens or whenever you experience synchronicity, *déjà vu*, a strange coincidence or any other type of dreamlike anomaly, take a moment to think, *That's weird. Could I be dreaming right now?*

Then perform a reality check (yes, in the waking state), and as long as your hand doesn't grow an extra finger or morph into a baby elephant, you can be sure that you're not dreaming.

Of course, I'm sure you know that you're not dreaming right now, but we're harnessing the power of habit. Doing reality checks in the daytime sets up a habit that'll crop up in your dreams, too, but in your dreams your hand *will* change and you'll become lucid.

Practise it every day if you can. Every time you see something weird or unexpected, notice it, ask yourself if you're dreaming and do a reality check. Most people find that they need to be doing 10 or more Weird Technique reality checks per day for the habit to enter into their dreams.

Charlie says

'The Weird Technique has 3 stages. Firstly, you acknowledge the weird or unexpected thing; secondly you ask yourself, "Could I be dreaming right now?" and finally you answer that question by doing your chosen reality check. Be sure not to miss out the second stage – this is the most important one and without it the technique won't work.'

Remember, by doing reality checks during the daytime, while you're awake, you're creating a habit that will then reappear in your dreams and lead to lucidity.

Professor Matthew Walker, author of the seminal book *Why We Sleep*, explains it like this:

> You start doing these checks throughout your entire waking day to the point where it becomes a reflexive habit, and then that habit bleeds through into your dreaming life from your waking life and you start to do the same reality testing in dreams. And at that point I think, 'Oh, the jig is up. I'm not awake. I'm dreaming.'[10]

Fascinatingly, lucid dreaming specialist Daniel Love has calculated that '11% of our mental experience each day is spent dreaming'.[11] He goes on to say, 'Just to clarify, this is not 11% of sleeping activity but 11% of your entire daily experience each and every day.'[12] This means that every time we apply the Weird Technique we have about a one in ten chance that we will actually be dreaming. I like those odds.

· ·

Let's Look for Weirdness!

In the waking state, whenever something strange or unusual happens, ask yourself, 'Am I dreaming?' and then answer the question by doing a reality check such as looking at your hand twice in quick succession or reading a piece of text twice in a row. If you do this 10 or more times a day, it seems to be enough for you to start dreaming about doing it and so lead to lucidity.

'As we live, so we dream', so don't just flip your hand over flippantly every time something odd happens, because that's what will happen in your dreams, too, rendering the technique useless. Be sure to act with full conviction and the expectation that the reality check will come back positive if you're actually dreaming.

Whenever you see something weird or unexpected in your daily life, take a moment to think, *That's weird. Could I be dreaming right now?*

Then perform a reality check. This sets up a habit that'll crop up in your dreams too.

The other option for using reality checks and the Weird Technique is simply to work on the basis of impossibility. During the daytime, anytime something weird or dreamlike occurs, try to do something impossible like breathing through your nose while pinching it or pulling your finger and making it stretch or jumping into the air and trying to float. In the waking state all of those actions will be impossible, but if you try to do them while you are dreaming, then you will actually breathe through your pinched nose, your finger will stretch when you pull it and gravity won't bring you back down to Earth.

· ·

Charlie says

'A woman on one my courses once said, "You want me to go around all day asking, 'Am I dreaming?' and looking at my hands to check if I'm awake? That'll send us all mad!" It's actually quite the opposite, though – every time we do a reality check we're practising sanity, because we're taking a moment to stop, come into the present moment and become more aware of our current reality.'

Pre-lucid Confabulation

Sometimes as beginners we might find ourselves in a dream, spotting a dream sign, about to become lucid... and then talk ourselves out of it. Other times we might become aware that we could be dreaming and do a reality check, but then become distracted by the dream before we can become lucid. This bizarre phenomenon is what I call 'pre-lucid confabulation'.

I was talking about confabulation at a retreat in Wales once when a psychologist in the audience said under her breath, 'You're bullshitting yourself.'

I stopped, looked at her and said, 'Excuse me?'

She replied, 'Confabulation is all about bullshitting ourselves. We bullshit ourselves in order to maintain the status quo of our reality. Psychotics do it all the time.'

It seems that when we are confronted by the possibility of recognizing that we're dreaming, our egoic sense of self often tries to confabulate a seemingly rational explanation with which to explain away the reality of the situation. For example, we might see a flying elephant in a dream and be on the cusp of lucidity, but then convince ourselves that flying elephants are quite common in this part of the world.

Why would our egoic sense of self do this? Because it feels threatened by lucidity. Once we're lucid, we see through the illusion of our egoic sense of self and become part of the dream, beyond any notions of 'me', 'my,' 'I' and 'other'. We are in fact one with everything in the dream and so the stranglehold of the egoic self is released. To prevent this, out of misjudged desperation it sometimes tries to prevent us from becoming lucid.

In the Castaneda text *The Art of Dreaming*, Don Juan tells his student that our rational mind will try to protect itself if we encounter ideas or concepts in our dreams that seek to usurp our notion of accepted rationality. This idea of rationality fighting for its own survival in the face of irrational dream experiences is one that beginner lucid dreamers may sporadically encounter, often in the form of dream characters denying that they are 'the stuff of dreams' as our rational mind tries to maintain control over the dreaming status quo.

Luckily, as our lucid dreaming practice progresses and our use of reality checks increases, the frequency of confabulation decreases, but beginners, beware: once you suspect that you might be dreaming, don't accept any facts to the contrary without checking them thoroughly. Just like Lieutenant Columbo.

The Columbo Method

No reality-check technique works 100 per cent of the time, so what do you do if you're in a dream, see a dream sign and do a reality check, but your hand doesn't change? How can you do the reading-text reality check if there isn't any text to read in the dream? How can you spot a dream sign if the dreamscape is seemingly devoid of them?

Sometimes you might find yourself in a scenario where both recognition of dream signs and reality checks seem null and void and yet you still have a gut feeling that you might be dreaming. This is when you need to rely on checking the facts and looking closely at your surroundings, like a detective scanning a crime scene. This is the basis for the Columbo Method.

For those of you old enough to remember him, think back to the 1970s TV detective Lieutenant Columbo. He was a cigar-smoking LAPD detective who represented every man's (and woman's) bumbling inner detective. Columbo didn't have flashy forensics or complicated theories, he just used his own sound judgement and awareness to detect the reality of a situation.

Columbo could walk into a room and notice 10 clues before he'd even introduced himself; he had a broad awareness that took in every detail of the environment while he remained totally relaxed, not giving anything away, just innocently puffing on his Cuban cigar. That's just how we need to be if we want to solve the mystery of the lucid dream.

Let's Search for Clues!

Once you suspect that you might be dreaming, look for evidence of dreaming just like a detective searching an area for clues. Be mindful, be aware, be vigilant. Try asking yourself, 'How did I get here? Where was I before I arrived here?' and 'look for rifts in cause and effect… and any impossibilities',[13] which will help you detect the dream state. Scan the area for clues, touch things, engage the space, be mindful. The dream state looks amazingly realistic, but if you look closely enough, you'll be able to see the inconsistencies and recognize that you're dreaming.

While you're searching for these clues, try to stay totally cool and calm, just like Columbo, because if you get overexcited, you may either wake up or give the game away, leading to the possibility of confabulatory new dream material that will uphold the illusion of the dream.

To really empower the Columbo Method, practise it in the daytime, too. We dream as we live, so as you go through your daily life, or perhaps for a designated 10 minutes a day, look very closely at things, feel the textures around you, investigate odd-looking places and examine your experience in depth. You can even ask yourself, 'How did I get here?' at regular intervals throughout the day.

If you do these types of engaged mindfulness practice often enough in the day, you'll end up doing them in your dreams, too.

Charlie says

'Now that we've covered a few techniques, you might be wondering what pace to take things and how long to spend on each one before moving on to the next. Check out the Creating a Practice section (see page 171) for tips and guidance.'

Mindfulness Meditation and Flow States

'Just mindfulness. If you train in mindfulness
you will surely recognize the dream.'[14]
Akong Tulku Rinpoche

Our final daytime techniques to explore are mindfulness meditation and flow states.

Mindfulness Meditation

Although the jury is out on whether mindfulness meditation actually increases the frequency of lucid dreams, it definitely helps to stabilize them and has a whole range of daytime benefits too.

The essence of mindfulness meditation is 'knowing what is happening while it is happening without judgement',[15] so lucid dreaming isn't just analogous to mindfulness meditation but is actually a direct extension of it. Lucid dreaming requires a constantly vigilant mindful awareness that has to be maintained throughout the dream, which is exactly what is required in waking mindfulness practice.

The dream yoga masters tell us that lucid dreaming is dependent on our ability to maintain focused awareness and the ability to 'hold one's mind in check'[16] as we sleep, two qualities directly fostered by mindfulness meditation.

Mindfulness is all about awareness. By training ourselves to be more aware, we naturally become kinder and happier, because almost all of our unkindness, to ourselves and others, stems from a lack of mindful awareness. It is said that 'in a state of mindfulness, you see yourself exactly as you are. You pierce right through the layer of lies that you normally tell yourself and you see what is really there.'[17]

Training ourselves to be more mindful is one of the greatest gifts we can give ourselves and others, but we don't just learn this by sitting down to meditate. Through lucid dreaming and conscious sleeping we can develop our capacity for mindful awareness while we sleep.

Daytime mindfulness has long been known to lead to mindfulness during dreaming. What is less known is that it works the other way around, too. Dr Akong Rinpoche, the man who co-founded Samye Ling, the first Tibetan Buddhist centre in the West, told me how this process worked. Usually a man of few words, he described in detail how lucid dreaming actually helped to strengthen waking-state mindfulness: 'Dream yoga is about mind training. It is about how not to lose your mind during sleep and is used to train the mind to maintain its all-round capacity for mindful awareness.'[18]

Some people think that meditation is about stopping thoughts, letting the mind go blank or having ecstatic experiences, but mindfulness isn't like that, it's simply about being aware of what is happening in our mind, without preference or judgement.

Any form of mindfulness meditation practice can be used to help fill the lucidity tank, but if you don't have a regular meditation practice already then you might like to try the wonderfully concise mindfulness exercise based on the Mindfulness Association UK's 'Settling, Grounding, Resting with Support' technique (see *the sitting meditation, page 249*).

Flow States

Although mindfulness may not actually lead to an increased frequency of lucid dreams, there is something similar to mindfulness that does.

Research from Maria Kozhevnikov, PhD, at Harvard has shown that people who regularly engage in activities that bring them into a flow state tend to have more lucid dreams.[19]

Following on from the well-established findings that video-gamers have more lucid dreams than the general population, Dr Kozhevnikov found that it was the psychophysiological arousal or 'flow' state that gamers were entering into while playing video-games that was the active ingredient in inducing more frequent lucid dreams.

The term 'flow state' describes a mental state in which a person is completely focused on and deeply immersed in a single task or activity, perhaps even experiencing a loss of awareness of themselves and a distorted sense of time. They may also report not thinking about the task they are doing but instead simply doing it.

Informally referred to as being 'in the zone', flow has similarities with mindfulness, but crucially, flow is an active state of psychophysiological arousal in which the subject is actually doing something. Rock-climbers, musicians, dancers, martial artists, extreme-sportspeople, video-gamers and artists often experience flow states when they are engaging in their practice.

Dr Kozhevnikov's research found that frequency of flow-state experience directly correlates with the frequency of lucid dreams. People who engaged in more flow-state activities had more spontaneous lucid dreams. So let's add dancing, rock-climbing and surfing to our toolbox of lucidity techniques!

Charlie says

'Dr Kozhevnikov's research ties in beautifully with the fact that meditation practices that contain an element of autonomic arousal and "flow-state" experience, such as Sufi whirling, Tibetan Buddhist tummo (inner heat) and Taoist tai chi have been known for thousands of years to help induce lucid dreams.'

CHAPTER 7

LUCIDITY IN ACTION: TOP 10 DREAM PLANS

*'We may judge of your natural character
by what you do in your dreams.'*

Ralph Waldo Emerson

Before we move on to the night-time techniques, I want to offer you my personal Top 10 favourite dream plans, because, as I said before, the 'why' is more important than the 'how' and dream planning is the most important technique there is.

When we find ourselves fully lucid within the amazingly realistic three-dimensional dreamscape of our own mind, the question of what to do becomes limited only by our imagination and the strength of our friendship with our unconscious mind. For those of you interested in the practice of dream yoga, this is really where the path starts in earnest.

Our level of volitional influence over our lucid dreams will increase with practice, and with sustained training we can get to a level where we can literally do anything our unconscious allows, without any constraints from the laws of physics. Certain activities may seem more difficult to engage in than others, but this is due to the limits of our expectations rather than the limits of the dream. The dream is limitless.

Remember, though, that once lucid, your actions at least directly affect your brain chemistry and at most actually rewire your neural connections, so choose wisely when deciding how to spend your lucid dreams.

When engaging intentional action in the lucid dream, the most important thing to remember is that manifestation follows thought, or, as the Buddha said, 'With our thoughts we make the world.' Robert Waggoner comments, 'The dream space largely mirrors your ideas, expectations and beliefs about it,'[1] so have full confidence that your *sankalpa* will be heard and that your dream plan will manifest.

Of course there are countless activities you can get up to in your dream world, but here are my personal Top 10 lucid dream activities, which I can say for sure can be of both psychological and spiritual benefit and also a whole lot of fun. I've used many of these dream plans with my own lucid dreams, which you will find in a section at the back of the book.

Here they are in roughly ascending order…

Number 10: Life Rehearsal

Coming in at number 10 is using the lucid dream for rehearsing new mental habits and letting go of doubt.

In the lucid dream you can work on aspects of your own psychology in a totally safe virtual reality of your own creation. If you are a painfully shy person, for example, you can use a lucid dream to practise being more outgoing by interacting with the dream characters. Whatever change you want to make in the waking state can be started in the safety of a lucid dream – a laboratory of change in which mistakes can be made and new perspectives explored without fear of failure.

One of the people who completed the 100-hour Lucid Dream Facilitator Training with me is a Somatic EMDR facilitator called Laura, who used lucid dreaming to integrate her stage fright.

She told me, 'I gave up doing live concerts around 13 years ago, because I felt so bad on stage it just didn't make any sense at all to continue. Emotionally, I was still stuck in a trauma response and just could not sing anymore.'

She created a dream plan to address this issue in which she would practise singing in public. In the dream she found herself in a pub, did the Columbo Method, became lucid and engaged her dream plan. She began singing to all the customers, playfully singing for each person and getting right up close to them, singing loudly and with joy. Her dream ended with her hugging one of the women she had sung for and telling her, 'From now on I will sing with peace and joy in my heart.'

Soon after this, the waking state presented her with a great synchronistic opportunity as she was asked to sing live on stage for the Christmas show at her daughter's school. Singing in front of all the pupils, families, friends and teachers was something that she would usually have refused, but she found herself happily agreeing. When the day came, she said she not only had zero anxiety, but had a huge desire to sing.

She told me, 'As I was singing, I couldn't help smiling: for the very first time in 13 years I was enjoying it! I could have sung forever! I wished it had lasted longer, and even when I walked away from the stage, I kept on singing happily. I felt so happy and grateful and relaxed. This possibility of using lucid dreaming to change what had seemed impossible to change, it really felt like magic!'

. . . .

Let's Rehearse!

Make a dream plan of practising a new skill or habit and then, once lucid, simply practise that skill or habit, just as you would when awake, but free from the waking state's limitations.

Once lucid, you may find yourself, as Laura did, in a space where you would normally perform this action, but it's not essential. It's more important just to carry out the dream plan – and to be mindful of the feelings and sensations that occur while you're doing so. These will reappear like real-life memories when you next perform the action in the waking state.

. . . .

Number 9: Asking 'Big Questions'

In at number 9 is using the lucid dream to ask big questions such as 'What is the nature of reality?' or 'What career path should I take?' or 'How can I be of most benefit?'

Your big question might be something personally significant or globally significant, but whatever it is, make sure that you really want to hear the answer that your dreaming mind will offer.

The library of enlightened knowledge that we all possess can often seem quite inaccessible in the waking state, but through lucid dreaming we gain access to it much more easily, and perhaps even access to the collective wisdom beyond the dream.

If we use the metaphor of the mind as an iceberg, which, as we know, is much bigger below the surface than it is above it, we can see that when we direct a big question to our unconscious mind within a lucid dream, the answer will come not just from the top 10 per cent of the iceberg (as it tends to when we're awake), but from the real powerhouse of the unconscious mind that forms over 90 per cent of our psyche.

The first time I tried this dream plan, I decided to aim high. I became lucid and yelled out to the dream, 'What is the essence of all knowledge?' The answer I received revealed both the wisdom and the sense of humour of the unconscious mind. (*For a full description of this dream, see Dream 7, page 265.*)

More recently I asked, 'How can I be of most benefit?' and the answer that I received led not only to reaching thousands of new students, but also gaining thousands of air miles. (*For a full description of this dream, see Dream 18, page 281.*)

My friend Nina asked, 'What shall I do career-wise?' and was shown an image of herself teaching kindergarten-age children. In the waking state she realized that this was something that she had actually always thought of doing and she subsequently went into training and has now been a primary school teacher for over eight years.

Another friend asked, 'How can I be of most benefit?' and the entire dream turned into symbols of love, with helium balloons in the shape of hearts and the word 'love' appearing everywhere in the dreamscape.

The options are endless and the answers you get can be life-changing.

Oh, and finally, if you can't think of a specific question or you simply want to see what your Dreamer has to offer, just call out, 'Show me something important!' or 'Show me something I need to know.' I used this dream plan a couple of years ago and my Dreamer presented me with the personification of Time, who gave me a crash course in how time works. (*To read the whole thing, check out Dream 17 on page 280.*)

Let's Ask a Big Question!

Make a dream plan of the question you intend to ask and then take a few moments to affirm your intention. Let your Dreamer know that you are looking to it for insight and guidance.

In your next lucid dream, simply state your question out loud to the dreaming mind – call it out to the sky or an open space rather than address it to a specific dream character.*

The reply you get may be as obvious as an immediate audible response from the dream or from a dream character, or as subtle as a symbolic change to the dreamscape, so make sure that you keep your senses engaged, ready to receive your answer in whatever form it may come.

Charlie says

'When I first started teaching at the age of 25, I really doubted whether I was qualified to teach dream work as a career. I felt too young and inexperienced to have much to offer. After a couple of years of wrestling with this, I had a lucid dream in which I asked for some career advice. My dreaming mind encouraged me to follow my dreams. It was one of the most important lucid dreams of my life.' (For a full description of this dream, see Dream 11, page 270.)

---

* If you pose your question to a specific dream character, the answer you get may be limited by your unconscious assumptions about that particular dream character, so it is far better to pose your question to the dreaming mind itself.

Number 8: Receiving Teachings

Rolling in at number 8 is receiving teachings. As I mentioned earlier, lucid dreams can be the medium through which we can receive teachings from our own innate wisdom essence, sometimes called our Buddha nature or higher self. But perhaps we can receive teachings from sources outside ourselves too?

The dream yoga teachings state that lucid dreams can be an excellent medium through which to receive spiritual teachings from the mindstream of enlightened masters, and some lamas even advise us to actively seek out such teachings by getting lucid and going to other realms of existence 'to study and see the teachers who live in these holy places'.[2]

Sometimes teachings will come to us without a request being made at all. To receive these teachings, the most important thing is to maintain a non-preferential openness to whatever our innate wisdom mind presents us with, because often the teachings will come to us in a way that we don't expect.

But we can also hasten the process by becoming lucid and calling out, 'Inner guru, come to me!' or 'Higher self, give me guidance!'

Sometimes the teachings that I've received in a lucid dream have been so precise and so seemingly unknown to me that I've found myself opening up to the possibility that they have been sourced from something outside my own personal mindstream. We can never know for sure, but if the teachings we receive are based on kindness and compassion, then maybe it doesn't matter where they're from anyway.

I once called out in a lucid dream for Lama Yeshe Rinpoche to give me teachings, and the detailed specifics of the advice he gave me really made me think that they might have been sourced from his mindstream rather than mine. (*For a full description of this dream, see Dream 4, page 261.*)

Let's Receive Teachings!

Make a dream plan to receive teachings and then, once lucid, call your *sankalpa* out loud to the dream, saying something like: 'Inner guru, come to me!'

If you have a link to a spiritual teacher, you can also call for them to offer you teachings. If they arrive and start teaching you, remember they may be just a mental projection or an actual aspect of that teacher. Only you can know for sure, but it is said that the inner guru is the ultimate teacher, so be grateful for either!

Number 7: Letting Go of Grief

We can also use lucid dreaming to meet dead people, whether mental projections of them or actual aspects of their spirit, and let go of grief.

I can almost hear the tuts of the sceptics as I write this, but please just do a reality check and hear me out. I'm not necessarily talking about communing with ghosts here, more about exorcizing the ghosts of the relationship we had with those we have lost or letting go of the grief that still haunts us.

We can use the hyper-realistic virtual-reality simulation of the lucid dream state to say a final goodbye, to ask for forgiveness, or to have one last hug with our deceased loved ones as a way of integrating grief and letting go.

In my second book, *Lucid Dreaming Made Easy*, one of the case studies is my friend Millie, who used to be a pole dancer and used a lucid dream to meet her dad, who died when she was 12. She had always carried some guilt about how he would feel about her chosen profession, and in the lucid dream she asked him about this.

He replied, 'Yes, I know everything that goes on, Millie, and I'm very proud of you all.'

Millie told me, 'The lucid dream was a way for me to get his blessing on how I live my life. He seemed so accepting and wasn't judgemental at all. He loved me regardless, and when I woke up, I was able to let go of my own judgements and know that he loved me whatever path I might take.'

I believe that it was letting go of her own judgements that was the real breakthrough. The important thing here is not whether Millie actually met the spirit of her dad 20 years after his death or whether it was simply a mental projection of him, but that she received the blessing of her inner father: that was where the real healing lay. To have her symbolic internal father archetype accept her fully created a powerful shift in her own self-judgement – a perfect example of how this technique works regardless of whether it's actually the spirit of the dead loved one that we meet or not.

Although I do believe that most of the time it is probably just a mental projection of the dead person, sometimes it may not be. I think there are some rare cases in which we may actually be contacting an aspect of the dead person's mindstream. From a Buddhist point of view, the mind of the 'bardo being' during the 49-day after-death *bardo* period is said to be nine times as powerful, meaning that whenever anyone thinks of them or says their name, they can hear it and are drawn instantly to that person. (This is why offering candles and prayers to dead people during this period is so important.)

So, if the *bardo* being has nine times the power of consciousness and the lucid dreamer has seven times as much, if we can connect with the *bardo* being within that 49-day period, the possibly of actually connecting with their mindstream is drastically increased. In fact, this means that the lucid dream state can be regarded as one of the most effective mediums for engaging in communication with dead people.

Charlie says

'You might be thinking, OK, so I get the 49-day thing, but what about those who died long ago? I asked Rob Nairn about this once and he told me that our ancestors could leave "a shroud of habitual patterns that survives after death" – an echo of their energy, with which we can sometimes communicate long after they've died.'

In the past nine months I have been able to put this to the test, as I lost my mum and my Buddhist teacher Rob Nairn within a few months of each other. In both cases, I was unable to have any dreams with them during the first few weeks, but at around the 25-day mark, in both cases, I became lucid and met them. I have no proof that it was actually them rather than my projection of them, but both of the lucid dreams were deeply healing. I was able to call out my mum's name and she appeared, looking in perfect health and much younger than when she died, and with Rob Nairn I found myself sitting at his feet, and when I asked him for 'one final teaching', his reply was unforgettable. (*For a description of this dream, see Dream 21, page 285.*)

Let's Let Go of Grief!

Make a dream plan for meeting someone you are grieving for and then take a few moments to affirm your intention.

In your next lucid dream, simply call out for the dead loved one, and whatever appears, whether a mental projection of them or an actual energetic aspect of them, send them love, say goodbye or do whatever you have decided you need to do in order to let them go.

Charlie says

'It is said in the teachings that if you are ever lucky enough to meet a bardo being, whether in a lucid dream or not, then it's just as important to assure them that they are dead as it is to tell them that they are loved. Until they can accept that they are dead, they may not be able to move fully through the after-death process. There are three vital points to tell them: you are dead, everything you are experiencing is mind, and go towards the brightest light you can see.'

Number 6: Doing Things That Scare You

In the Tibetan dream yoga teachings of Guru Padmasambhava, he speaks of four stages of dream yoga.[3] The first stage, 'recognition', is simply about becoming lucid, but the second stage, and thus the first thing we are advised to do once lucid, is to engage with the 'transmutation' of fear and the release of the energetic blocks it so often creates.

We do this by intentionally doing things that scare us, such as 'jump from a high place, knowing that you cannot die' and 'walk into fire, knowing that you cannot be burnt'.[4] We are even told to call a tiger into the dream so that we can 'jump into its mouth, ride on its back and even make friends with it'.[5]

This training in fearlessness doesn't just affect our dream life, it affects our waking life too. The Tibetan dream yogis say that when we become aware of our dreams, we will start 'waking up to our delusory thoughts while we are awake... we will stop being duped by our projections'[6] and be less afraid of living our lives fully and joyfully.

It even helps us at death too. If we can train in fearlessness in our dreams, we can create a habit of courageous calm that will be a huge benefit to us in the after-death states. Lama Yeshe Rinpoche once told me, 'In dreams, your fear can become 100 times more powerful, but in death it can become 1,000 times more powerful! We must train in fearlessness in our dreams to prepare to be fearless in death.'[7]

So I advise you to use your lucid dreams to do things that scare you, because, as the great 10th-century female Buddhist master Machig Labdrön said, we should 'go to the places that scare us in order to find the Buddha within'.[8]

Let's Do Scary Things!

Create a dream plan around the fear you wish to face and then, once lucid, simply engage in the fearful activity, reminding yourself at all times that you are dreaming and so your body is safe in bed.

Although the Tibetan teachings encourage us to 'call forth a tiger' or 'jump from a high place', I would ask you: 'What is your tiger?' Perhaps it is fear of rejection or childhood trauma? 'What is the high place from which you fear to jump?' Perhaps it is stepping into your power or making a shift in your life.

Number 5: Walking through Walls

The third stage of dream yoga is called 'multiplication' and involves exploring the empty nature of the dream state.

Back in Chapter 4 we explored how the Buddhist term *shunyata*, 'emptiness', actually meant pure potentiality and how something empty of inherent existence could contain infinite possibility. In the lucid dream state we can experience emptiness directly, because we can see how everything that seems real and solid is just a projection of our own mind, totally impermanent and brimming with infinite manifestations.

The Tibetan dream yoga teachings advise the lucid dreamer to explore the seemingly solid appearance of the illusory dreamscape as a way of appreciating the dreamlike nature of waking reality. They also actively encourage us to 'multiply' the dreamscape we are exploring: 'If the dream be of minute objects, transform them into large objects' and 'If the dream be of a single thing, transform it into many things.'[9]

However, I have found that one of the best ways to explore the concept of emptiness within a lucid dream is to try to walk through a wall. This is a way not only to gain ultimate insight into the illusory nature of dream projections, but also to systematically train the mind to break through the habit of viewing solid things as impenetrable. The esteemed dream yogi Namkhai Norbu Rinpoche says that if we can use the lucid dream state to 'pass through seemingly solid walls, this is a very favourable experience for overcoming the attachments of daily life, because we experience directly the insubstantiality and unreality of all things'.[10]

Charlie says

'Rob Nairn once told me, "It's only doubt that stops us walking through walls, Charlie."[11] I agreed and started telling him about a lucid dream in which I got stuck halfway through a wall because I had a moment of doubt. He looked at me, smiled and said, "I wasn't talking about lucid dreams, I was talking about real life."'

I was first instructed to 'walk through walls'[12] in a lucid dream by the late, great Buddhist teacher Akong Tulku Rinpoche, and the first time I tried it, the wall was totally solid and I hit my face on it and woke up.

The next time I tried it, I stood in front of a wall, fully lucid, reminded myself of the empty nature of the dream state and that in the dream the wall did not exist. Then I did actually manage to move through it as it became soft like liquid concrete until halfway through, when I had a moment of doubt and the wall resolidified around me. My doubt created the resolidification of the illusion.

Upon the third attempt I became lucid and with full confidence called out, 'I'm dreaming, this is all an illusion empty of inherent existence! The wall does not exist, everything is mind!' before running through the wall successfully. (*For a full description of a wall-walking dream, see Dream 14, page 276.*)

What an amazing teaching Akong Rinpoche had given me through those three words: 'Walk through walls.' In fact, the real teaching came in the waking state, when I realized that every time we walk through a wall in a lucid dream, we are engaging a new mindset that says, 'What seems to be solid is not always so.' And with that, we are empowered to walk through the brick walls of our own bullshit in the waking state too.

....

Let's Walk through Walls!

Once lucid within a dream, find a wall, remind yourself that it is actually a mental construct with no solidity at all and then try walking or running through it.*

Some people like to wade into the wall very slowly, experiencing fully the sensations of solidity or liquidity, while others like to run full pelt into the wall so that the experience is over as quickly as possible! There is no 'best practice' as far as this is concerned.

---

* It's common to feel some physical resistance while passing through an object. This is the ego-mind trying to maintain the usual illusion of solidity. Just remind yourself, 'This is the stuff that dreams are made of.'

False awakenings are a common occurrence with this technique, so be sure to do a reality check straight afterwards.

Charlie says

'Every time we walk through a wall in a lucid dream we are creating a new habit, a new neural pathway in our brain. This new pathway says, "That which seems solid is not always so." Cultivation of such a revolutionary new habit affects our waking life in that we come to see emotions, prejudices and fears as similarly unsolid.'

Number 4: Physical Healing

Hitting our chart at number 4 is one of my all-time favourite applications of lucid dreaming: physical healing. To engage this technique, all you require is some sort of physical ailment that you would like to heal.

The esteemed dream researcher Jayne Gackenbach, from Virginia University in the USA, cites examples of lucid dream healing of everything from nicotine addiction and hives to weight loss. In my second book, *Lucid Dreaming Made Easy*, I include a case study in which a man with kidney disease did hands-on healing within the lucid dream and his kidneys stopped deteriorating and his creatinine level remained stable for nine months afterwards. I have healed everything from addictive behaviour to ear infections through this method, so it doesn't matter what the ailment is, only that you have the strong belief that you can heal it through lucid dreaming.

Rosanne, another of the Lucid Dream Facilitator trainees, used lucid dream healing to rehabilitate her knee. She says, 'I raised my left hand to the sky and called forth the healing energy: "Healing energy, come to me." I lowered my hand to behind my left knee, and a burst of white light was emitted. That surprised me – a sign that the dream was doing its own thing. Then I said, "My knee is free from pain," once and, "My knee is free from inflammation," three times. The next morning the pain was completely gone and I could walk perfectly.'

As we learned earlier, whether the Tibetan Rinpoches are right about the 'seven times the power of mind' or not, a very powerful placebo effect can definitely be engaged through lucid dreaming.

Buddhist scholar B. Alan Wallace says, 'It should be called the mind effect, not the placebo effect! It's all about the mind affecting the body.'[13]

The lucid dream is a state of pure mind and so the 'mind effect' works with maximum efficacy when engaged within it.

Add to this the fact that, as we learned in Chapter 1, once lucid, the brain thinks we are awake and will rewire itself in response to any lucidly dreamed activity, and we can see why lucid dream healing can work so effectively for some people. Some but not all, of course. Lucid dreaming isn't a silver bullet, and for every amazing story of healing that I have heard there are probably 100 failed attempts that I haven't heard about. However, the worst that can happen is nothing, so it's well worth a shot.

- -

Let's Heal!

Make a dream plan for your intended healing.

Once lucid, if you wanted to heal your ear, for example, you could apply hands-on healing within the lucid dream and imagine coloured healing light surrounding the area, while calling out statements of healing intent such as, 'My ear is healed! My immune system is boosted!'

This three-step protocol of hands-on healing, healing light and affirmations of healing is a pretty good one to follow, but if the manifestation of healing light is a bit too tricky, then just state out loud your healing intent, for example, 'I am free of any and all non-beneficial disease' or 'I am healed of my toothache' while directing healing intent to the area of disease or discomfort by placing your hands on the affected area within the dream.

And finally, to send healing to another person, either invoke a visualized projection of them within the lucid dream and apply hands-on healing or simply call out statements of healing intent for them. Rest assured, if the healing isn't for their highest benefit then it simply won't affect them, so the worst that can happen is nothing.

Charlie says

'I had heard of loads of people healing physical ailments through lucid dreaming, but I had never experienced it first-hand. That was, until I contracted an ear infection from surfing and proceeded to heal it in a lucid dream!' (For a full description of this dream, see Dream 16, page 279.)

Number 3: Inner Child Healing

We learned earlier that we all have an inner child, an archetypal representation of our connection to childhood, and that not only the health of our inner child, but our development as a human being is greatly impacted by the experiences of the early years of our life.

The qualities of a healthy inner child are often listed as wonder, joy, optimism, playfulness, curiosity and spontaneity. These are all true, but we must remember that the inner child is also strong:

they survived. They are still here, and so they are a source of strength too.

Lucid dreaming is one of the most direct ways to access this strength. Pioneer of inner child work the late Cathryn L. Taylor believed that it was through the personification of the inner child that the most powerful healing could be accessed, because it allowed us to relate to a representation of our childhood in a tangible manner. I believe that this is what makes lucid dreaming such an effective way of working with the inner child, because in a lucid dream the inner child will literally be personified.

In 2023, I used inner child healing to integrate the grief of my mum's death. She died after a gruelling seven-year battle with early-onset Alzheimer's disease, and one of the unique aspects of Alzheimer's is that it gives you two deaths: the physical death and the psychological death, the death of the personality, which often happens years earlier. For me, this meant that when my mum physically died, I didn't actually feel that heartbroken by it, because my heart had been broken three years earlier, when she had died psychologically and forgotten who I was, lost the ability to speak and stopped being able to mother me. That's when I felt that I had really lost my mum.

But to my inner child that wasn't the case. Although my adult self seemed OK when she died, 'Little Chuck' wasn't. He had just lost his mummy and he was grieving and sad and angry.

It was fascinating to see this show itself in my waking life through flashes of childlike rage and in my dreams as terrible nightmares of grief so deep that I would wake wailing like a toddler. My Dreamer, that part of the mind that creates and plays out our dreams, was doing what it does best: highlighting the inner wounds that I was ignoring in my waking world.

So I made a dream plan to heal my grieving inner child and as soon as I became lucid, I called out, 'I love you, inner child, I love you!'

Then I asked for my inner child to actually appear, and when he did, I began hugging him lovingly. As I hugged him, a feeling of bliss erupted into the dream, and along with the euphoria was a feeling that I hadn't felt for many years: it was something similar to the feeling of believing in Santa Claus, an intense feeling of childhood magic. (*For the full dream, please see Dream 20, page 284.*)

After that lucid dream, the moments of waking rage stopped and the grief nightmares soon faded away. Something had shifted within me.

Let's Heal the Inner Child!

Make a dream plan to heal your inner child and then, once lucid, simply call out statements of healing, such as, 'I love you, inner child! I heal my inner child' or an invocation to meet the inner child, such as 'Inner child, come to me!* I want to meet my inner child!'

And whatever appears, whether a personification of the inner child or a cloud of energy, embrace it with love.

If it was blame and shame that wounded your childhood psyche, you might like to also call out statements such as: 'It wasn't your fault! You are such as good little boy!'

As with all of these Top 10 dream plan suggestions, these are simply suggestions, so absolutely make them your own and use whatever affirmations feel best for you.

---

* I believe that the first act of both reparenting your inner child and showing them your love is to give them a name they love, so feel free to use a childhood nickname or a name that you wished you had been called as a child when you call for them.

Number 2: Integrating the Shadow

Almost at the top of the chart we find lucid dream shadow integration. As mentioned in Part I, the shadow is the part of us that is made up of all that we hide from others: our shame, our fears and our wounds (the dark shadow), but also our divine spirit, our blinding beauty and our hidden talents (the golden shadow).

The dark shadow is often misinterpreted as some sort of evil or demonic presence that is both separate from us and harmful to us, leading us to waste the valuable learning process it offers us by investing our energy in ways to defeat it. The truth is that the shadow is neither external nor harmful. It isn't an entity that has entered our dream, it isn't an external demon that a shaman has sent into our mind, it's the amalgamation of the wounded and rejected aspects of ourselves. It is our 'dark side', but not dark meaning 'evil', but dark meaning 'yet to be illuminated'. As Jung commented, 'In spite of its function as a reservoir for human darkness – or perhaps because of this – the shadow is the seat of all creativity.'[14] It is part of us, and until we accept that its darkness doesn't come from an external 'evil' but from a wellspring of internal creativity, we'll never be able to be a fully integrated human being.

David Richo, in his brilliant book *Shadow Dance*, describes the dark shadow as 'a cellar of our unexamined shame' and the golden shadow as 'an attic of our unclaimed valuables'.[15] Shadow integration involves shining a light into the dark caves of our dreaming and waking minds to reveal the gold that is stored there.

Although it seems obvious why we would hide our dark shadow from others, why would we hide our golden one? We are often just as scared by the brilliance of our divine light as we are of our darkness. Through lucid dreaming, we can face and embrace both our dark and golden shadows in personified form.

In lucid dreams, a dark shadow aspect may take form as obviously as a nightmarish monster rampaging towards us or as subtly as a dream character who is just particularly repellant, and the golden shadow might appear as a divine being or a power animal, but whatever form the shadow takes, rather than running from it or feeling scared by it, we should actively embrace it with the compassionate realization that it is merely a mental construct that we now have the valuable opportunity to integrate. Actively embracing it might mean something as literal as hugging it or as subtle as turning and facing it with acceptance and courage. It's about doing the opposite of what we usually do when we meet our shadow, which is to turn away from it.

I've been hugging shadow aspects for almost 20 years now, and in my 2011 TED talk I talked about the first time I did so and how the shadow monster transformed until I was literally hugging myself.[16] And in my shadow integration book, *Dreaming Through Darkness*, I include a dream from a Christian friend of mine who became lucid in a nightmare in which a demon was chasing him and he realized that this demon must be a shadow aspect, so he decided to confront it. He asked it, 'What do you represent?' And in a deep, booming voice, it replied, 'I am your sin!' Without missing a beat, he hugged it with love, and although it initially struggled in his embrace, it dissolved into light and disappeared.

If you can literally embrace your shadow with love in a lucid dream, then, as a Jungian psychotherapist who was on one of my retreats said, 'You can integrate as much shadow material in one lucid dream as in six years of therapy!'

Charlie says

'Shadow integration is one of the most powerful psychological healing techniques available to the lucid dreamer. In just one lucid dream we can make strides towards healing and integration that might have taken years in the waking state. We can directly converse with personified shadow aspects and even dissolve them into our own dream body as a symbol of full integration.' (For a full description of this practice, see Dream 6, page 263, and for another great shadow integration dream, see Dream 5, page 262.)

Let's Integrate the Shadow!

The fundamental way to practise dark shadow integration in lucid dreams is that whenever we encounter a frightening, perverted, violent or distasteful dream character or dream scenario, we should actively embrace it with love, rather than either running away or rejecting it through violence.*

For golden shadow integration it's the same, but the golden shadow will often be less obvious, appearing as a spiritual being, sexually liberated person, amazing singer or the embodiment of whatever gold within yourself that you refuse to acknowledge.

In the first edition of this book I only offered one option as far as meeting your shadow was concerned, but over the past decade I've seen that there are loads of options:

- You could call out to meet your sexual shadow: the personification of everything that you have rejected, denied or disowned pertaining to your sexuality.

---

* Shadow integration and fearlessness in dreams may naturally start to manifest in our waking world, too. We begin to see aspects of our own negative projections that we can integrate, just as we have trained to do in the dream.

- You could ask to meet your teenage shadow: the embodiment of everything you have rejected, denied or disowned pertaining to your teenage years.

- You could call out to meet your golden shadow: all the divine, untapped potential within you that you dare not acknowledge.

- For a brilliant start to your shadow work you could just call out a more general, 'Shadow, come to me!', in which case it will most often be some sort of representation of your dark shadow (perhaps the psyche initially prioritizes this integration over that of the golden shadow?)

Whatever appears, give it a hug and show it love. Doing this may well be the single most important thing you will ever do.

Charlie says

'Please note that if you call out, "Shadow, come to me!" in a lucid dream, you'd better be ready for it, because you've just opened the floodgates and called forth the totality of both your darkness and light! Although this technique is absolutely safe (and in fact the shadow will only present you with what you are ready for), I advise that you try it only when you are feeling grounded.'

Number 1: Meditation and Spiritual Practice

At number 1 in my Top 10 chart we have meditation and spiritual practice in the lucid dream! This can be a truly powerful experience and it's my all-time favourite thing to do once lucid.

As I mentioned earlier, in the waking state our spiritual practice is often hindered by the limitations of our physical body and the flow of our *chi*, but in the lucid dream state we are unhindered by these limitations and can consequently reach levels of meditation which far surpass our waking practice.

Opposite, we will learn how to do a Tibetan Buddhist dream yoga practice as an extra bonus technique, but this number-one slot is absolutely not just for those into Buddhism, but for people of all traditions and none. If you are a shamanic practitioner, call your power animal into the lucid dream, if you're a Christian, then commune with the spirit of Jesus, if you are a mindfulness practitioner who uses a meditation app on your phone, then do that mindfulness practice within the lucid dream.

And if you don't currently have a spiritual practice to do, then do the original spiritual practice: send love and healing to others.

Simply saying a few prayers within a lucid dream or meditating for a few seconds has immense spiritual benefits, because, as we learned earlier, just one moment of spiritual practice in the lucid dream state is worth a one-week meditation retreat in the waking state.

Let's Do Spiritual Practice!

Once you are lucid, engage in your spiritual practice. Whether it's mindfulness meditation, mantra recitation or saying prayers of healing, just carry out the practice in roughly the same way as you would in the waking state.

Remember, though, that in the lucid dream you don't need a meditation cushion or prayer beads or a temple – wherever you are when you become lucid, just get straight into it.

Meditation in lucid dreams can often lead to incredibly strong sensations and experiences, so the most important thing is to stay grounded in the awareness that it is all a fabrication of mind.

> **Charlie says**
>
> I've had loads of experiences of meditating in the lucid dream state, but one of the most profound was actually when I tried it for the first time. I was only 19 years old and I didn't really know what I was doing. It totally blew my mind, and when I woke up, I felt as if a curtain had been lifted.' (For a full description of this experience, see Dream 2, page 258.)

Bonus Practice: Chenrezig Dream Yoga

I was in two minds about whether to include this practice at all, let alone put it as a bonus practice, but I decided that it was too beneficial to leave out.

Although this is a full-on Tibetan Buddhist dream yoga practice, and so perhaps more relevant to Buddhist readers, it includes a mantra said to 'liberate all who hear it',[17] so reciting this mantra just once in a lucid dream is a very beneficial thing to do, whether you're a Buddhist or not, and can lead to powerful spiritual experiences.

Many of the Tibetan Buddhist dream yoga practices require a qualified lama to teach them and a set of initiations to receive them. But this one can be both shared and practised by everyone. It is the practice of Chenrezig.*

Chenrezig (Sanskrit: *Avalokitesvara*) is the buddha of infinite compassion. In fact, we may do better using the term 'universal archetype of compassion' instead, as an archetype is a primordial principle that exists in each one of us, but also exists independently.

Chenrezig is depicted as sitting cross-legged and having four arms, representing loving-kindness, joy, compassion and equanimity. He wears a crown and certain ornaments, all of which have specific

---

* In his book *Living, Dreaming, Dying* Rob Nairn clearly states, 'People who can dream lucidly but have not been initiated can visualize the embodiment of compassion, Chenrezig, and recite the associated mantra in their lucid dreams.'

meanings (see page 59 for the image), but essentially this archetype is the essence of universal love and compassion in personified form.

Each deity in Buddhism has a certain mantra associated with them, and for Chenrezig it's the well-known: *Om mani padme hung* (Sanskrit) or *Om mani pemé hung* (Tibetan).

We could dedicate a whole chapter to the meaning of this mantra, but the best explanation I've ever heard is 'love in the form of sound'.

Charlie says

'The word "mantra" gets thrown around a lot nowadays, but what does it actually mean? Man in Sanskrit means "mind" and tra means "that which protects", so we could say that a mantra is a series of sounds, syllables or words that have a protective effect on the mind.'

Essentially, this dream yoga practice is based around three steps once we become lucid:

1. mantra recitation

2. deity visualization

3. self-visualization as the deity

The fruition of many waking-state Tantric Buddhist practices is self-visualization – using your imagination to transform yourself into the deity or archetype that you are working with. In the lucid dream state this self-visualization actually becomes self-manifestation, because the imaginary realm of the lucid dream state allows visualization to manifest into form. This is extremely beneficial for our spiritual development and leaves a powerful energetic imprint on our mindstream.

Within the lucid dream this self-visualization, or perhaps more accurately self-manifestation, as the deity is how we enter stage 4 of dream yoga: 'unification', in which we transform ourselves into the form of an enlightened being (in this case Chenrezig) as a way of unifying with its, and our, enlightened nature. This is the fruition of dream yoga practice.

This is also a great practice to help with the after-death *bardo*, because whatever we train to do once lucid, we will habitually do upon recognition of the death *bardo*. It is said that if we say the *Om mani pemé hung* mantra just once in the after-death *bardo*, we will be liberated into full enlightenment. In fact, I once asked Rob Nairn, 'What would happen if one were to think of Chenrezig as one were dying or in the after-death *bardo* states?' and, pausing for theatrical effect, as he so loved to do, he turned to me and said, 'If you were able to think of Chenrezig just once in the death *bardos*, he would appear before you, take you by the hand and guide you to the pure realms of enlightenment.'

Let's Do Chenrezig Dream Yoga!

- Once lucid, recite the mantra *Om mani pemé hung* out loud over and over again, with love and compassion.

Charlie says

'In the waking-state practice of Chenrezig, the visualization usually comes before the mantra recitation, but due to the stabilizing qualities of mantra on the mind, I usually recommend lucid dreamers to start with the mantra and then try the visualization.'

- Then, if possible, visualize Chenrezig in the space in front of you. (*Use the image of Chenrezig on page 59 to familiarize yourself with the image.*) Don't worry if you can't get it super-clear, and feel free to use a ball of compassionate white light instead if you like.

- Finally, see if you can merge with Chenrezig, either by bringing him into you and then transforming into him or by keeping the front visualization as it is while transforming yourself into him. This final stage is a powerful experience in which the aspiration is to literally transform into the deity, so that when you look down, you no longer see your body, but instead see the form of Chenrezig. This self-manifestation may be as a body of light, as if you are a hologram or movie projection. In this state, you spontaneously merge into the inseparability of your own enlightened nature.

But if this all sounds a bit complicated, just try saying *Om mani pemé hung* in the lucid dream. Doing this just once is one of the most incredibly beneficial things that you could ever do and will plant such a powerful seed of infinite love that your current life and all future lives will be beneficially affected by it.

· ·

CHAPTER 8

NIGHT-TIME LUCID DREAMING TECHNIQUES

*'First recognize the dream. Use anything that helps —
the techniques elucidated by the dream yogis or
any of the methods of modern lucid dreaming...
The whole point is to become lucid within the
dream so that you have the basis for whatever
dream yoga activities you choose to enact.'*

B. Alan Wallace[1]

Now that we've covered the daytime techniques, we're ready to move on to the techniques that we do as we are actually falling asleep. The following practices aim to train our mindful awareness during all stages of dreaming, sleep and the liminal spaces between the two. Rather than just focusing on lucid dreaming, we focus on strengthening lucidity in all states of consciousness, just as the original dream yoga teachings recommend.

By combining Western and Eastern night-time techniques, my aim is to take the ancient power of the Tibetan Buddhist approach to dream work and make it accessible to Western practitioners without any homogenization of the two traditions.

The Stages of Sleep

Having a basic knowledge of the stages of sleep is fundamental to understanding how and why the night-time techniques work. If we want to dream lucidly, we need to understand when we're most likely to be dreaming, so that we can schedule our lucid dreaming practice accordingly. So, here are the various stages.

Stage 1: The Hypnagogic State

This is the transitional state between wakefulness and sleep. In the hypnagogic, our eyes are closed and we feel very drowsy, but we haven't actually fallen asleep yet, so we can still hear the sounds in the room and still feel our body in the bed. For many, the most recognizable aspect of this 'doorway into sleep' is the hypnagogic imagery: the dreamy hallucinations, both visual and auditory, that flash and fade in our mind's eye as we drift off.

These psychedelic images are made up of memories of the day, mental preoccupations and the displays of our subconscious mind. While in the hypnagogic state, we might experience sudden bodily spasms, known as 'myoclonic jerks', which often become incorporated into hypnagogic 'micro-dreams', perhaps as stepping off a kerb or falling off a ledge. Some researchers believe this is an evolutionary throwback to when we used to sleep in trees – the jerk would help us maintain awareness of our sleeping place, so we didn't fall out of the tree. Others believe that it is the body's response to the steep drop in blood pressure that occurs when we pass through the hypnagogic unusually quickly, often due to overtiredness.

Neurologically, the hypnagogic stage of sleep is accompanied by alpha and theta brainwaves, which are associated with states of hypnosis and deep relaxation. This makes it a deeply suggestible state, which is why so many of the lucid dreaming techniques involve reciting affirmations in it.

Stage 2: Light Sleep

Following the half-awake/half-asleep hypnagogic state, we enter light sleep, where we experience the dissolution of external awareness and we black out. As we enter light sleep, our heart rate starts to drop, our body temperature lowers, our eye movements stop and our brainwave activity slows down.

Dreaming comes later in the sleep cycle, but if someone is woken from light sleep, they will often report thinking about something or exploring an idea.

Neurologically, light sleep is dominated by theta brainwaves, which are associated with flow states and meditation, interspersed with bursts of rapid, rhythmic brainwave activity known as sleep spindles. Although it may not seem the most exciting sleep stage, we spend more time in light sleep than in any other stage and it makes up about 50 per cent of our total sleep time.

Stage 3: Deep Sleep

As we fall further into slumber, our brain begins producing very low-frequency delta waves and we enter the deepest level of sleep. In deep sleep, our brain is highly deactivated, and if we are woken from it, we'll commonly feel groggy and disorientated. It is a restorative sleep stage in which our heartbeat and breathing slow to their lowest rates and we quite literally detoxify our brain through an increased volume of cerebrospinal fluid,[2] which flushes out neurotoxins, including a protein called beta amyloid that is linked to Alzheimer's disease. This process improves memory processing and consolidation, optimizes immune function and restores cell energy stores.[3]

As you can imagine, without deep sleep, our brain function is greatly impaired the next day. Deep delta-wave sleep is also essential for general bodily repair, as it's the state in which HGH, human growth hormone, is released. This makes our cells regenerate and our hair, nails and muscles grow. We get most of our deep sleep in the first four hours of our sleep cycle, which is why we can physically survive for quite a while on just four hours of sleep. But to thrive, rather than simply survive, it is essential to have the REM (rapid eye movement) dreaming sleep that follows it.

REM (Dreaming) Sleep

After a long chunk of deep sleep, our brain switches from its most deactivated state to a state that is even more active than waking: REM sleep. That is when we dream.

During dreaming, the mind is projecting dynamic three-dimensional fully operational worlds into which the dreamer is placed. This is a highly active neurological process that actually requires more brain capacity and cerebral blood flow than everyday wakefulness. Our dreaming brain isn't resting, it's working flat out to maintain the intricate projection of our dreaming reality, a projection often so realistic that most of us accept it as real every time we enter it.

We have our first dream period within about 90 minutes of falling asleep, and although we do dream throughout the whole night, the majority of our dreaming is done in the last few hours of an eight-hour cycle. Dreaming is an active sleep state – our brainwave activity, breathing and blood pressure all increase to near waking levels, while the actual process of dreaming requires so much neurological energy that it even burns calories. Our body doesn't move, though – it becomes paralysed so that we don't act out our dreams. A part of the brain called the pons sends a signal to the spinal cord to paralyse the major muscle groups.

As recently as a couple of decades ago the neuroscientific community was still unsure as to what the main purpose of dreaming actually was. But we now know that we dream in order to learn. Scientific research shows that 'REM sleep doesn't just hit the "save" button on memories, it actually hardwires them into the brain and then hits the "save" button.'[4]

Sleep expert Professor Matthew Walker famously stated: 'We dream to remember and we dream to forget.'[5] We dream to remember the details of experiences of the day that might help to further our future wellbeing and to forget (let go of or integrate) the traumatic or painful emotional charge of past experiences. Dreaming is just as essential to our health as neurotoxin-removing deep sleep. In fact, when we're sleep-deprived, our brain actually prioritizes dreaming over the other three stages of sleep.

The Hypnopompic State

The final sleep stage is more of a transitional state than a sleep-stage proper. It's the state of mind between sleep and wakefulness, the hypnopompic state. In this state, our eyes are still closed, but we can hear the sounds in the room and we're no longer asleep, but we're not quite awake either. Just as the hypnagogic is the doorway into sleep, the hypnopompic is the doorway out.

The Journey into Sleep

Sleep is a cyclical journey that progresses from hypnagogic drowsiness through light sleep, down into the depths of deep sleep and then up into the realm of dreaming every 90 minutes or so, multiple times throughout the night.

Our first dream period is only about 10 minutes long, and the whole cycle, from the moment of falling asleep to the end of our first REM period, usually takes about 90–120 minutes. We repeat this 90-minute cycle multiple times throughout the night, spending increasingly more time in REM and less time in delta wave as the night progresses. As our REM periods get longer, the last two hours of our night's sleep end up consisting of mainly REM dreaming. The REM cycle has grown from about 10 minutes to at least 45 minutes or more by the end of an average seven- or eight-hour sleep cycle.

It's worth mentioning that most of us have brief awakenings throughout the night, often at the end of each 90-minute cycle, but because we ordinarily don't have any memory of them, we think we've slept constantly. People with problematic sleep, however, tend to grasp at these micro-awakenings and panic, because of their hyperconscious fear of not being able to sleep when they 'should' be asleep. This reaction causes their brain to awaken even further and stress hormones to be released, and so perpetuates the cycle.

In 15 years of teaching workshops on sleep and dreams, I have yet to meet anyone who sleeps in a perfect four-stage 90-minute sleep cycle, so please use the information in this chapter simply as a rough framework for exploring how you sleep. Your aim here is to empower yourself with knowledge, not to get hung up on the fact that you may not sleep in exactly the same way as others.

The most important point for lucid dreamers to remember is that the first half of the night is mainly deep sleep with short dream periods and the second half of the night is when we have long REM dream periods with not much entry into deep sleep.

The last few hours of our sleep cycle is also when we will enter dreams most easily from the waking state. This makes it a prime time for lucid dreaming. While we can absolutely have lucid dreams in the first few hours of our sleep cycle, the dream periods will be shorter and our mind might not be as fresh. However, in the last few hours we will not only have longer dream periods, but also have a fair few hours of sleep under our belt, so our mind will feel fresh and be ready to engage lucidity.

From a Tibetan Buddhist perspective, it is said that clarity dreams (which include lucid dreams) occur more readily in the last two hours of our sleep cycle, so it seems that the last two hours of sleep are really the golden time for lucidity.

Charlie says

'Remember, although the majority of people sleep in this way, you may not be part of that majority. Some people have full-on lucid dreams within 30 minutes of falling asleep at night. We all sleep differently, so get to know the way that you sleep, not the way everybody else sleeps.'

The Clear Light of Sleep

Tibetan Buddhism agrees with the Western scientific view of the four stages of sleep, but the major difference is that the Tibetan tradition views dreamless delta-wave sleep as the most important stage, because it is here that we can experience the clear light of sleep.

One way that this occurs is when we become super-lucid within the dreamless delta-wave deep sleep state, entering into the state of mind beyond all aspects of subject–object dualism, which has been described by the great Tibetan scholar Patrul Rinpoche as 'the original state of the mind, fresh, vast, luminous, and beyond thought'.[6] The clear light of sleep is actually the pinnacle of all dream yoga practice and 'the closest we get to the enlightened mind, where the veils obscuring our enlightened nature are at their thinnest'.[7]

The concept of being lucid within the dreamless void of our own mind is difficult to comprehend and currently yet to be validated by science, but on the rare occasions that I may have stumbled into it, I've found it to be an infinite void of what I can only describe as a 'luminous darkness', or perhaps more fittingly as a 'dazzling darkness'[8] — a term the early Christian Gnostics used to describe ultimate reality.

So, now that we have an understanding of how our sleep cycles work, let's get back to learning how to become lucid through the night-time practices.

Hypnagogic Affirmation Technique

This practice is found in all the major dream traditions, from the Sufis to the Toltecs, the Buddhists to the shamans, and in all of them it follows a similar structure: waking in the second half the night and falling asleep again reciting an affirmation to gain lucidity.

All of these traditions knew that the second half of the night was where dreams could be accessed more readily and that the power of intention was king in the realm of lucid dreams.

As we've learned, the hypnagogic state is very similar to the hypnotic state, so if we apply a suggestion or affirmation within it, we may find that it has the potential to work with hypnotic effect.

I want to offer you four variations of this technique so that there is something for everyone, but if you want to create your own version of this practice, then please do so.

All the variations follow the same structure: you wake yourself after four or five hours of sleep, and then drift back to sleep while reciting an affirmation of lucidity. I suggest reciting your chosen affirmation at least 21 times in a row. This is a suggestion taken from the Tibetan Buddhist tradition, but is a pretty good recommendation across the board. Originally the Tibetan dream yogis would use their prayer beads to count their sets of 21 affirmations, but feel free to use your fingers instead.

Within the dream yoga teachings of the great master Guru Padmasambhava, it is said that you should 'bring forth a powerful yearning to recognize the dream state',[9] so you really need to make your intent to gain lucidity strong and real for any of these affirmations to work effectively.

Simple Affirmation

Let's begin with the simple version of the practice.

. . . .

Let's Do It!

- Set your alarm for about five hours into your sleep cycle.

- Wake up with the alarm, write down any dreams you remember and drop back into the hypnagogic state.

- Once in the hypnagogic, mentally recite: 'The next time I'm dreaming, I'll know that I'm dreaming' or 'The next time I'm dreaming, I'll remember to recognize that I'm dreaming,' or whatever phrase you feel best encapsulates your intention to get lucid, over and over, at least 21 times in a row if you can. There is no need to actually say the numbers in your head; use your fingers to keep count instead.

- After a few minutes of recitation, allow yourself to fall asleep with a mind saturated with the strong intention to gain lucidity. Or, if you still feel wide awake, do another set of 21 affirmations.

- Try to recite the affirmation with real gusto – this is vital, because without determination, this technique simply won't work.

. . . .

The Bodhicitta *Affirmation*

The second version of this technique comes from the Buddhist tradition and is based on the concept of *bodhicitta*. As we learned earlier, *bodhicitta* – 'heart of the awakened mind' or the 'spirit of awakening' – is about dedicating our actions to the benefit of all beings.

Bodhicitta lies at the core of every practice within the Tibetan Buddhist tradition, as it encompasses both the ultimate aim of reaching full enlightenment for the benefit of all beings and the relative aim of being kind and loving to all beings for the benefit of all beings.

So, the affirmation we use here is: 'I lucid dream for the benefit of all beings' or some people might prefer 'I recognize my dreams for the benefit of all beings' or maybe 'I lucid dream with the heart of awakening.'

It's said that when the buddhas and bodhisattvas, enlightened beings and deities, hear someone stating their intention to do something for the benefit of all beings, they gather round that person and support their endeavour. So, when you use this affirmation you get the back-up of the buddhas, which makes it very powerful.

. . . .

Let's Do It!

- Follow the same steps as for the Simple Affirmation (waking after five hours, diarizing your dreams and dropping back into the hypnagogic).

- Replace the affirmation with: 'I lucid dream for the benefit of all beings' or 'I recognize my dreams for the benefit of all beings.'

- Mentally recite it at least 21 times as you fall asleep.

. . . .

Charlie says

'If you're a Buddhist practitioner, feel free to create an affirmation containing the mantra of the particular deity or buddha with whom you feel a connection. For example, I like to use the mantra of Amitabha Buddha, Om ami dewa hri, as part of a rhyming affirmation: 'Om ami dewa hri, now I have a lucid dream.' This not only serves the purpose of the technique, but it also imbues the practice with the blessing of the mantra.

The Toltec Affirmation

The shamanic tradition of the Toltecs flourished in Mexico over 850 years ago and lucid dreaming was a key part of it. The Toltecs used certain breathing exercises before sleep to 'plant' dreams and to encourage lucid dreaming as well as using masks and obsidian mirrors to manipulate their reflection as a way of practising shape-shifting in lucid dreams.

My connection to this tradition is through my friend Sergio Magaña, author of *The Toltec Secret*, and it was he who taught me the affirmation that we will use in this version of the technique.

Similarly to the Tibetan Buddhist tradition, the concept of the 'spiritual warrior' was central to the Toltecs. In fact, lucid dreaming was often referred to as 'the warrior's path', not because you fight anything, but because it takes the discipline of a warrior to have a lucid dream. So in this version of the technique, our affirmation will be the Toltec affirmation 'I am a warrior of the dream state. I stay lucid and conscious while dreaming.'

At my workshops, this is often an affirmation that splits the group. Some people really connect with the idea of the dream warrior, while others find it a bit too 'yang' for their tastes. Give it a try, but only use it if you like it.

···

Let's Do It!

- Follow the same steps as for the Simple Affirmation (waking after five hours, diarizing your dreams and dropping back into the hypnagogic).
- Replace the affirmation with: 'I am a warrior of the dream state. I stay lucid and conscious while dreaming.'
- Mentally recite it at least 21 times as you fall asleep.

···

> ### Charlie says 💬
>
> 'The Toltecs and Buddhists have been using this technique for hundreds of years, so how did they wake themselves up without an alarm clock? The Buddhists just used the power of intention, while the Toltecs used a swig of fig wine before bed. It's a diuretic, so would make them wake up to pee after a few hours!'

The Dream Plan Affirmation

The fourth and final version of this technique is the dream plan affirmation. This is a great one to use if you are worried that you may forget your dream plan or *sankalpa*, because it uses an affirmation that references these.

Let's Do It!

- Follow the same steps as for the Simple Affirmation (waking after five hours, diarizing your dreams and dropping back into the hypnagogic).

- This time add your *sankalpa* to the affirmation or a few words that encapsulate your dream plan. For example: 'The next time I'm dreaming, I'll know that I'm dreaming. When I know that I'm dreaming, I'll… meet my inner child' or 'The next time I'm dreaming, I'll know that I'm dreaming. When I know that I'm dreaming, I'll… heal my sexual shadow.'

- Mentally recite it at least 21 times as you fall asleep.

Top Tips for All Variations

- You can do this technique as you first fall asleep at night, but for best results do it after an early-hours wake-up about five hours after you went to bed.

- If you are currently experiencing high levels of stress, anxiety or heartache, you may find that if you wake up, you may not be able to get back to sleep. If that keeps happening, then only practise this technique as you first fall asleep.

- The important thing is not so much that you're repeating the affirmation right up to the point at which you enter a dream (although that would be great), but more that you saturate your last few minutes of conscious awareness with the strong intention to gain lucidity.

- You should be mentally reciting your chosen affirmation for a minimum of 2 minutes and a maximum of 10 minutes.

- If you wake up to pee at nights, that gives you a perfect and non-disruptive chance to practise this technique as you fall back asleep. No need for an alarm clock!

LaBerge's MILD (Mnemonic Initiated Lucid Dream)

This is probably the best-known lucid dreaming technique in the West and is the technique Dr Stephen LaBerge developed that allowed him to have lucid dreams at will.

Mnemonic means 'pertaining to memory' and a Mnemonic Initiated Lucid Dream is one that works by using the function of memory combined with an affirmation similar to the simple one used in the previous technique. Many people find MILD to be one of the most effective lucid dreaming techniques there is.

The MILD technique is based upon the principles of visualization, autosuggestion (self-hypnosis) and prospective memory. Interestingly, the basis of the technique can be found as far back as the 16th century, but a full explanation of the modern version is given in *Exploring the World of Lucid Dreaming* by Stephen LaBerge.

Although visualization and autosuggestion provide the foundational power of this technique, it is prospective memory that provides the real crux. We use prospective memory all the time in daily life when we say things like 'Next time I see a bank, I'll remember to get out some cash.' And it's actually a very reliable aspect of memory.* If we use it with strong intent, we activate the motivational or goal-seeking part of the brain, which will stay unconsciously activated throughout both waking and sleep states until that goal is achieved. In the same way, a prospective memory command that we set as we fall asleep, such as 'Next time I'm dreaming, I'll remember to recognize that I'm dreaming,' will stay neurologically engaged until we next find ourselves dreaming.

MILD is a technique that requires us to visualize ourselves back in the dream that we were just having and so is best practised after waking from a vividly recalled dream. This can be done naturally, perhaps when you've woken up in the early hours, or intentionally, by setting an alarm to wake yourself up during a REM period sometime in the last few hours of your sleep cycle.

Charlie says

'Are you worried that all this waking up with alarm clocks could make you feel less rested? Remember, restorative sleep occurs in deep delta-wave sleep during the first four to five hours of sleep, whereas these lucid dreaming techniques are practised in the last few hours of sleep and, crucially, during REM sleep, when the brain isn't resting anyway.'

---

* If you've ever set a strong intention to wake up at a certain hour and succeeded, then you've used exactly the same 'goal-seeking' neurological activation that the MILD technique employs.

Let's Get MILD!

Step 1: Recall the dream

- After awakening from a period of dreaming, wake up fully and recall the dream that you were just having. If possible, find a scene or part of the dream that had a dream sign in it. Memorize this particular part of the dream. (You'll find out why in step 3.)

Step 2: Set the intent

- Now get ready to go back to sleep. As you begin to fall asleep and enter the hypnagogic state, mentally recite over and over again, with determination and enthusiasm: 'The next time I'm dreaming, I'll remember to recognize that I'm dreaming.' Focus on this command and if you feel your mind wandering or realize that it has wandered already, just bring yourself back to the recitation. Totally saturate your mind with the intent. This is the all-important prospective memory and autosuggestion part of the technique and its effectiveness depends on imbuing the recitation with wholehearted 'joyful effort'.*

Step 3: Visualize lucidity

- Once you've created and stabilized the strong motivation to *remember to recognize that you're dreaming*, the next step is to visualize yourself back in the dream sequence or scene that you recalled earlier. Really try to relive it in as much detail as you can, envisaging yourself back in it and experiencing it with all your senses as you drift off to sleep. However, this time, imagine that you recognize that you're dreaming and become fully lucid. How? By imagining yourself spotting a dream sign, and then having the realization *Aha! I'm dreaming!*

- Then imagine calling out to or engaging your *sankalpa*.

---

* One of the Buddhist six perfections, 'joyful effort' is the term used to describe enthusiastic effort in spiritual practice.

The two core principles of the technique are engaging your prospective memory with strong intent and then visualizing yourself getting lucid.

The combination of imagining becoming lucid in a recent dream scene, while in a state of self-hypnosis, and while reciting a lucidity affirmation, creates a very powerful technique.

Step 4: Drop off to sleep or do it again

- Now you can either just fall asleep or repeat steps 2 and 3 (set the intent and visualize lucidity) until you feel sure that you've fully engaged the technique, at which point you can allow yourself to fall asleep.

Charlie says

'An easy way to remember the order of this technique is like this: M-I-L-D: M = Memorize the dream you were just having; I = set the Intent; L = visualize Lucidity; D = Drop off to sleep or Do it again.'

The 'Wake Up, Back to Bed' Method

This technique was first posited in the late 1970s by G. Scott Sparrow, the author of *Lucid Dreaming: Dawning of the Clear Light*, and is one of the most effective lucid dreaming techniques available. In fact, Buddhist scholar B. Alan Wallace references research that calculates that this method increases your chances of lucidity by a whopping 2,000 per cent.[10]

So, how do you practise this seemingly too-good-to-be-true technique? It's simple. Wake up about two hours earlier than normal, stay awake for about an hour and then go back to sleep for another hour or two. Research shows that 'wakefulness interjected during sleep increases the likelihood of lucidity'[11] and that this technique is one of 'the most powerful, promising means of achieving lucidity, with over two-thirds of participants recording lucid dreams under these circumstances'.[12]

One of the ways this technique works is by harnessing the phenomenon of REM rebound. This phenomenon is based on the fact that if a person misses a whole night's worth of REM sleep, their next sleep cycle will contain much more REM in order to 'pay back the debt' from the previous night.

The last two hours of our sleep cycle are when we do most of our dreaming, so if we starve ourselves of this dream time, when we do eventually go back to sleep, we 'rebound' rapidly into vivid REM sleep. As REM sleep is the playing field for lucidity, we can see how this technique opens up the potential for getting lucid.

Feel free to experiment with waking three hours earlier rather two hours earlier, if you prefer, and with staying awake for between 30 minutes and 90 minutes, if you prefer.

And to really super-charge this technique, recite one of the variations of the Hypnagogic Affirmation as you fall back asleep.

Let's Wake Up and Go Back to Bed!

- Set your alarm for about two hours earlier than your usual wake-up time.

- Wake up, write down your dreams and get out of bed.

- Stay awake for about an hour, engaging in any fully wakeful activity. Meditating or reading about lucid dreaming is ideal, but I've found that just about any mindful activity works well. The aim is not to stay drowsy for the 60 minutes but to waken fully – full wakefulness being a prerequisite to the technique's efficacy. Having said that, drinking double espressos or answering work e-mails might arouse you a bit too much, so be mindful to keep sleep within arm's reach.

- After about an hour, reset your alarm for an hour or two later, return to bed and fall asleep again with the strong intention to gain lucidity.

· ·

Charlie says 💬

'All the other night-time techniques can be practised every night, but Wake Up, Back to Bed should only be attempted two or three times a week. This is because it is dependent upon a slight disruption of the sleep cycle, so if you do it too often, your sleep cycle will simply adjust to the change and the technique might stop working so well.'

FAC (Falling Asleep Consciously)

This practice combines elements of the well-known Wake Initiated Lucid Dream (WILD) technique with a few of my own adaptations and a twist of Buddhist mindfulness. Its aim is to enter REM dreaming sleep without blacking out or losing conscious awareness. It is both incredibly simple and often incredibly elusive, letting your body and brain fall asleep while your mind stays aware.

The efficacy of this technique, like so many, depends on when you do it. If you wanted to enter the dream state consciously from your first descent into sleep at night, you would need to maintain conscious awareness for about 90 minutes throughout all the stages of sleep that precede it.

Retaining one-pointed awareness for 90 minutes into sleep is a pretty tall order – in fact, the Dalai Lama says that 'going through this transition [from wakefulness into sleep] without blacking out is one of the highest accomplishments for a yogi'.[13] Luckily, there is a way that we can cheat a little bit…

If we practise this technique after briefly waking in the last couple of hours of our sleep cycle, we will enter REM dreaming straight from the hypnagogic state rather than having to go through the whole sleep cycle again. This means that we can enter REM dreaming within about 15 minutes, which is much more realistic length of time to stay conscious for and an accomplishment that even L-plate dream yogis can achieve.

For now, we'll explore three of the best variations of this technique.

Hypnagogic Drop-in

To enter the dream state lucidly, be like a surfer. Paddle through the hypnagogic imagery and 'drop in' to the wave of the dream lucidly.

• •

Let's Drop In!

- Sometime after at least five or six hours of sleep, wake up fully and write down your dreams. Then set your intention to gain lucidity, close your eyes and allow yourself to drift back into sleep.

- As you enter the hypnagogic, gently focus your mental awareness on the hypnagogic imagery and simply paddle through it, allowing it to build, layer upon layer.*

- The key here is to maintain a delicate vigilance without losing consciousness and being sucked into the dream state unconsciously.

---

* Depending on the time of night and varying from person to person, sometimes the hypnagogic doesn't actually contain much hypnagogic imagery. In that case, simply use the Body and Breath technique (*see page 147*) instead.

- Try to 'lead your mind delicately into the dream state like leading a child by the hand'.[14]

- Don't engage the hypnagogic imagery that will arise, but don't reject it either, just lie there watching it until the dreamscape has been formed sufficiently for you to drop into it consciously.

- If you feel yourself blacking out, just keep bringing your focus back to the hypnagogic state. The imagery and feeling of the hypnagogic is your mindfulness support and is used to keep the thread of your awareness engaged while the rest of you falls asleep.

- The hypnagogic imagery will continue to build layer upon layer until it starts to coalesce into an actual dreamscape. This is a wonderful thing to witness. It's a bit like watching dough rise and eventually become bread. It moves from a liquid, doughy state into the solid bread state quite rapidly. (*Check out Dream 19, page 283, for a good description of this process.*)

- As the dreamscape solidifies, you might feel a slight pull or sensation of being sucked forward. This is an indication that the wave of the dream is now fully formed. In surfing terms, you are on point-break.

- If you can just stay conscious for a few more moments and be ready to take the plunge, you'll find yourself dropping into the wave of the dream with full lucidity.

Charlie says

'This technique is just like surfing – it's all about persistence, balance and patience. Just as we harness the power of the wave to move along it, so we harness the power of the hypnagogic. Once we drop into the wave, we don't try to overpower it, we learn to utilize its power to experience something beyond ourselves. It's just the same with dreaming.'

Body and Breath

However far out your mind may seem to go during sleep, there are two aspects of your being that remain in your bed: your body and your breath. In waking meditation we can use our body and breath to anchor our awareness so that our mind stays stable and is less likely to lose itself in distraction. This is exactly what we want to do as we slip into dreaming.

Let's Do It!

- Sometime after at least five or six hours of sleep, wake up fully and write down your dreams. Set your intention to gain lucidity, close your eyes and allow yourself to drift back into sleep.

- As you enter the hypnagogic, gently focus your awareness on the sensations of your body and the breath flowing through it.

- Hypnagogic imagery will still arise, but rather than focusing on it, focus on your bodily sensations and your breathing. You might find that a systematic scanning of your body works well for this while slowing down your breathing. Alternatively, you might choose to simply allow your bodily sensations to command your attention as they arise. Becoming aware of the contact points of your body on the bed works well.

- Once you have scanned your body or become aware of particular sensations, become aware of your whole body as it sits in space. Hold your entire body within your awareness.

- At some point you may actually feel the body paralysis that accompanies REM sleep setting in. This means that you are at the doorway of dreaming.

- If you feel yourself blacking out, just keep bringing your focus back to the sensations of your body and breath. Use these to hold your awareness.

- By anchoring your awareness in this way, you will be able to float through the hypnagogic stage with conscious awareness and enter the dream state with full lucidity.

Counting Sleep

By combining counting with constant reflective awareness as you go through the transition from wakefulness into dream consciousness, you can maintain your awareness fluidly. This technique is much less meditative than the last two, but is just as effective and some people get the hang of it a bit more easily.

Let's Do It!

- Sometime after at least five or six hours of sleep, wake up fully and write down your dreams. Set your intention to gain lucidity, close your eyes and allow yourself to drift back into sleep.

- As you enter the hypnagogic, continuously reflect on your state of consciousness as you count yourself into dreaming, mentally asking yourself, for example, '1. I'm lucid? 2. I'm lucid?' and so on.

- For the first few minutes the answer each time will probably be: 'No, I'm still awake!', but once you've counted into the twenties, the answer will probably be: 'No, but I'm now in the hypnagogic!'

- If you can make it into the thirties or forties or even fifties without blacking out, the answer may become: 'Almost! The hypnagogic is starting to solidify. I can feel the dream coming!'

- Of course the eventual aim is to answer the question with something like: '61. I'm lucid? Hang on. Yes, I'm dreaming! I'm lucid!' as you find yourself fully conscious within a dream.

The Multiple Wake-ups Technique

The theory behind this technique is that if we only fall asleep once a night and then wake up once in the morning, we're only giving ourselves one opportunity to engage lucidity. That's just one opportunity to fall asleep consciously, one opportunity to recall our dreams and one opportunity to engage in lucid dreaming techniques. But if we wake ourselves up and fall back asleep three times a night, we triple our potential success rate!

On the lucid dreaming retreats that I run we have our first wake-up about five hours after going to sleep and then do two or three more alarmed wake-ups 90 minutes or so thereafter.

The first four to five hours of sleep are when we get most of our deep restorative sleep, so we don't interrupt that, but the second few hours, as you'll remember, are when we start to have longer dream periods, with the last two hours of our sleep cycle being the prime time for dreaming. And if we time the wake-ups to coincide with our ascent to the upper regions of sleep (which occur at the end of every 90-minute sleep cycle), we will still feel quite well rested the next day.

The multiple wake-ups technique has been used by Tibetan dream yogis for hundreds of years and in the dream yoga teachings of Namgyal Rinpoche we are actually instructed: 'Instead of a long continuous sleep, try to sleep for short periods by deliberately waking yourself up in order to review whether you have successfully recalled or recognized your dream.'[15]

Let's Do it!

A typical night-time schedule on one of my lucid dreaming retreats goes like this: after an initial period of about five hours of sleep alone in our beds (three 90-minute cycles plus 30 minutes leeway), we wake up and go to the meditation hall, where we have a 'sacred sleeping area' set up. Then, once we are side by side with our fellow dreamers, the night progresses in 90-minute sessions interspersed with periods of about five minutes or so for dream documentation. Although this practice greatly increases the chances of having a lucid dream, if you feel like these wake-ups will negatively impact your sleep too much, then feel free to skip it.

Feel free to adapt the schedule below to suit your personal sleep cycle and waking times. Experiment with two-hour sessions rather than 90 minutes if you prefer, and see what works for you.

- 11 p.m.–4 a.m: First session of sleep and dreams, focusing on restful deep sleep rather than any dream work *per se*.

- 4 a.m.–5.30 a.m: Second session of sleep and dreams, with specific lucid dream induction methods (e.g. the MILD technique).

- 5.30 a.m.–7 a.m: Third session of sleep and dreams, with specific lucid dream induction methods (e.g. the Hypnagogic Affirmation technique).

- 7 a.m.–8.30 a.m: Fourth session of sleep and dreams, with specific lucid dream induction methods (e.g. the FAC technique).

This schedule gives you over nine hours of sleep and triples the chance of getting lucid each night. This is due to the wake-ups, of course, but also due to the full nine hours of sleep. Crazy as it may sound, seven hours of sleep gives us just half the dream time of nine hours. This is because dreams tend to come towards the end of the night, so staying in bed an extra hour or so will make lucid dreaming much easier to achieve.

You might even like to think about setting up your own sacred sleeping area in your home. The simple act of dividing your sleep into a period of rest in bed followed by a period of spiritual practice (in a place other than your bed) creates a powerful energetic intention that directly translates into lucidity.

Please don't try this technique every night. On the four-day lucid dream retreats we offer optional night-time wake-ups every night, but this is only for a few nights and under retreat settings. Maybe just try it once a week or once every two weeks.

Maintaining Lucidity

Have you ever been to the circus and looked up at the tightrope-walker balancing on the high wire, unfazed by the huge drop either side? Maintaining lucidity is just the same in that it's about balance. On one side of the lucidity tightrope there is non-lucid dreaming and on the other side there is the waking state. Just as a novice tightrope-walker might only be able to take a few steps at first and stay on the wire for just a few seconds, so a novice lucid dreamer might only be lucid for a few brief moments. But with sustained practice we will eventually be balanced up on the wire for as long as we wish – maybe even doing backflips along it!

For many beginners, the difficulty is not so much getting on the lucidity spectrum as staying there. The 'Aha!' moment of lucid awareness is often followed by a rush of adrenaline that can be so strong that we lose our balance and fall off the tightrope into the waking state. The first few realizations of 'I'm lucid! I'm actually lucid!' can be so exhilarating that we can find ourselves awake in our bed, still buzzing with excitement, before we have actually had time to engage in any lucid exploration.

On the other hand, we can fall the other way, into non-lucid dreaming. This is usually caused by becoming distracted and forgetting that we're dreaming. Our attention is often diverted by some bizarre or attractive element of the dreamscape. This is like the tightrope-walker who spots a waving child in the audience below and, in that split-second of distraction, slips and falls off the tightrope.

The Tibetan masters advise us that we should extend the periods of lucidity for longer and longer, so we should really try to keep our balance on the lucidity tightrope for as long as possible. Don't forget, the lucid dream state is a more refined level of consciousness, so every second of lucidity is beneficial and healing for our mind.

There are loads of techniques for maintaining lucidity, but here are a few of my favourites, which I've found can maintain lucid awareness for extended periods of time. In fact, using these techniques I have even been able to maintain lucidity throughout an entire 60-minute REM period.*

'Keep Calm and Carry On!'

Older readers may remember the famous slogan of the British Home Office that encouraged Londoners to 'Keep calm and carry on' during the bombing raids of the Second World War. We need to 'keep calm and carry on dreaming' in order to avoid the panic of waking up when the bombs of distraction start falling.

The first part of this technique is simply to apply whatever we would do to keep calm in the waking state to the lucid dream state. Once we realize that we're lucid, we might feel the tightrope start to wobble a bit, but if we actively try to keep calm and mentally stable, we should be able to regain our balance. For me, this usually means talking to myself, saying, 'OK, Charlie, keep calm. It's all a dream. Keep calm.' For others, it might mean regulating their breathing or self-soothing in some way.

---

* As we learned before, estimation of time in the lucid dream state is the same as in the waking state. So if it feels as though you've been lucid for 10 minutes, you probably have been.

The second part of the technique is to 'carry on', because if we stay too still or prevaricate about what we want to do, we may find that lucidity begins to slip. Fortunately, calling out our *sankalpa* and engaging our dream plan is a great way to 'carry on' and will often immediately stabilize the dream.

Lucidity Boost

If we feel the sense of lucid awareness start to fade, we can enhance our lucidity by calling out loud within the dream, 'Lucidity boost!' or 'Amplify lucidity!', which will lead to an increase in lucid awareness as well as a sharpening of detail in the dreamscape.

I know this sounds crazy, but it seems that while we're lucid dreaming, an aspect of our mind sometimes called the 'conscious-unconscious', or what I refer to as The Dreamer, is aware of what we are doing and so can increase lucid awareness upon command. The command is at its most impressive just at the point at which the lucid awareness is fading, but it can also be used right at the start of the lucid dream as a way of increasing clarity and mental focus.

Give and Take

If you want to maintain lucidity for extended periods of time, you need to maintain a delicate balance between objective detachment and subjective participation. You have to be aware of the dream, but also totally aware that it is a mental projection that you are dreaming into existence. Too much detachment from the dream and you may fall into a semi-lucid state or simply wake up. Too much over-engagement in the dream and you may slip into the all-encompassing self-identification that characterizes non-lucid dreams. Too much control and The Dreamer may eject you from the dream, too little and you might not be able to engage your dream plan. Active participation is vital to engage the full potential of the dream and to maintain the awareness that 'because this is my dream, I can influence it', but too much and we may forget that 'everything I am experiencing is the dream and I am just one part of it.' On the tightrope of lucidity, balance is key!

Arm Rubbing and Hand Checking

This technique isn't hard to explain: if your lucidity starts to slip, begin rubbing the arms of your dream body and/or perform hand reality checks. This is not only a great way to remind yourself that you are still dreaming (due to the hand reality checks), but it's also a great way to bring your attention back to the somatic awareness of your body.

Your body is likely to be one of the few constants in the lucid dream – while the dreamscape may be morphing around you, your body will probably remain unchanged. By bringing your awareness back to your body, you bring your mind back into check.

The dream yoga teachings say that one of the reasons that you wake up from a lucid dream is that you start to re-identify with your physical body in bed, and so to counteract this, you need to identify fully with your 'dream body' by looking at it and touching it.

Spinning

This is a classic LaBergian technique used to maintain lucidity and simply consists of spinning around in your lucid dream. It works by harnessing the vestibular system of balance, which is found in the inner ear and not only helps to integrate information about bodily movement into the neurological system (which creates our visual experience of the world), but is also linked to the rapid eye movements of REM sleep.

It seems that the act of spinning around in a lucid dream tricks the mind into activating the vestibular system just as it would if we were spinning while awake, and this helps to maintain REM sleep and thus the stability of the dream.

. . . .

Let's Spin!

- If the visual dreamscape in your lucid dream begins to break up or fade and you feel yourself losing lucidity, stretch out your arms* and spin around like a whirling dervish. As you do this, the dreamscape will often blur into a haze of motion or fade to black.

- While you are spinning, hold the intention: 'The next thing I see will be the reformed dreamscape' or 'I am spinning in order to maintain lucidity.'

- After you have spun around for a few rotations or when you feel confident that you have set your intention strongly enough for the technique to work, stop spinning and you should find yourself in either the same or a newly formed dreamscape with full-level lucidity.

It should be noted that spinning can often lead to a false awakening (dreaming that you have woken up), so be sure to do a reality check immediately after this technique.

. . . .

As we come to the end of our night-time techniques section, it's worth saying that all of these techniques require sustained practice in order to work, but as long as we're applying them with the correct motivation, lucidity will surely manifest.

---

* Just to clarify: In bed, your sleeping body is paralysed by REM sleep and totally still, but in your dream you are spinning around like a spinning top.

As the Tibetan Buddhist nun Thubten Chodron says, 'When you plant seeds in the garden, you don't dig them up every day to see if they have sprouted yet. You simply water them and clear away the weeds; you know that the seeds will grow in time. Abandon impatience and instead be content with creating the causes... The results will come when they're ready.'[16]

CHAPTER 9

LIMINAL STATE TECHNIQUES

*'Relax but do not fall asleep, and be in a state
of awareness for as long as you can.'*

Don Juan Matis, Yaqui Indian sorcerer[1]

Now that we've covered both the daytime and night-time lucidity techniques, we'll be moving on to the practices of the liminal states – the meditative sleeping practices that involve maintaining lucid awareness through the gateways into and out of sleep. These practices not only directly benefit your lucid dreaming but are also brilliant stand-alone techniques.

The Hypnagogic and Hypnopompic States

As we discussed earlier, the hypnagogic state is the transitional state that lies between wakefulness and sleep. It is the dozy in-between state often characterized by hypnagogic imagery – the visual or often conceptual displays that flash and fade before our mind's eye as we drift off to sleep. These hypnagogic hallucinations are made up of memories of the day, mental preoccupations and, for some people, a whole load of crazy shapes, colours and faces. I imagine these eccentric displays of mind as a bit like the flashes of colour that you see during the final moments of a sunset, and, just like those final moments, they offer us a rare glimpse of our own inner light.

At the other end of sleep we find the hypnopompic state, which is the transitional state that lies between sleep and full wakefulness. Most people hardly even notice the hypnopompic state, because they pass through it so quickly in their rush to wake up. If only we spent more time exploring it, we would find that it's a state often characterized by flashes of inspiration and non-judgement as our mind rises afresh out of the darkness of sleep. I call these flashes of clarity 'hypnopompic insights'.

The hypnopompic is most commonly experienced as the half-sleep state that we enter after we've hit the alarm clock's snooze button in the morning. It's the state that we experience just before our mind has woken fully from sleep and when our eyes are usually still closed. It is a subtler state than the hypnagogic and contains much less mental imagery, as it's a state of mind in which we are partially awake but are yet to engage in fully conscious thinking.*

The unique feature of the hypnopompic is that because it occurs *after* a period of sustained sleep and dreaming, it is a much more refined state of mind, due to the psychological processing that occurs during sleep and dreaming.

The hypnagogic is of course characterized by drowsiness, because we are falling asleep, while the hypnopompic is characterized by a soft clarity of mind, because we have just been refreshed by sleep but aren't yet fully awake.

As we learned earlier, mindfulness meditation is about 'knowing what is happening as it is happening', so hypnagogic and hypnopompic mindfulness techniques are about knowing what's happening as it's happening *while we're dozing or snoozing*.

How do we actually do it? Let's zzzzzzzzzzzzzzzzz...

---

* This doesn't mean that there aren't thoughts in the hypnopompic, but we are much less likely to *engage* those thoughts with our chattering conceptual mind.

Hypnagogic Mindfulness (The Tao of Dozing)

We pass through the hypnagogic state every time we fall asleep, which means that we have a daily opportunity to engage it with awareness and even engage mindfully the sleep that it leads us into. It's a state of huge potential, but how can we spend more time in it than the 10 or so minutes that it usually takes to fall asleep? We must learn the Tao of Dozing…

With practice, we can literally meditate into sleep, which, as the Buddhist master Mingyur Rinpoche said, 'will mean that the sleep mind forms out of the meditation mind, which will make the sleep a meditation'.[2]

If we can practise mindfulness within it, the hypnagogic state can contain riches that will make us feel as though we've been sleeping on a goldmine for our whole life but have never gone digging.

This technique is about learning to rest on the drowsy boundary of sleep. The key to it is to be fully aware of the process of falling asleep so that we can begin to slow it down, giving ourselves extended access to the hypnagogic state and even bringing our awareness into sleep with us.

This practice is very similar to Yoga Nidra, but it's self-guided rather than audio-track guided, as many Yoga Nidra practices are. It's a form of mindfulness meditation that follows the 'Settling, Grounding, Resting' protocol taught by the Mindfulness Association UK.

And because it follows a mindfulness meditation format, it has the same amazing neurological benefits as standard mindfulness meditation, such as an increase in the grey-matter density of the hippocampus (an area responsible for learning and memory) and decreased density in the amygdala (an area responsible for anxiety and stress responses),[3] as well as all the benefits of NSDR (non-sleep deep rest) and Yoga Nidra.

This practice can be done at night as a precursor to sleep, but is best learned and explored during the daytime, when we are less likely to fall into full sleep. If we practise it during the day as an alternative to an afternoon nap, we may find that it refreshes our mind even more effectively than napping. It's a bit like putting the computer into 'hibernate' mode rather than 'shut down' mode: we save our battery power, but don't take so long to boot back up again.

And of course it's the perfect training for all those lucid dreaming techniques that require us to stay conscious in the hypnagogic while we are reciting our affirmations.

Let's Doze!

Prepare your space. This practice can be done sitting upright in a relaxed position, but ideally you should be lying down comfortably, usually on your back, either on the floor, on a sofa or in your bed. Most people like to have a pillow under their head and some people have a pillow under their knees, too, to help relieve lower back pain. You want to feel totally comfortable, so use as many pillows, blankets and supports as you need. Unless you are doing this practice as a precursor to sleep, you don't want to be so comfortable that you black out instantly, though, so be mindful of that.

Do whatever needs to be done to allow you to relax easily and then read through the following instructions to roughly memorize the different stages of the practice.

If you aren't using the practice as a precursor to sleep, set a gentle-sounding alarm for 20–30 minutes later.

- Close your eyes and relax.

- Become aware of your breathing and then settle your mind by breathing in for a count of three or four and breathing out for a count of three or four.

- Continue breathing this way for a few minutes. When you have thoughts, just let them go freely, without attempting to reject or engage them. Simply leave them be and bring your focus back to the breathing and counting.

- After a few minutes, begin to focus a little more on your out-breath. Notice that as you release it, your body relaxes a little more.

- And then feel free to drop the breath-counting.

- Now, breathing naturally, begin to ground yourself by bringing your awareness into your body. Simply become aware of all the bodily sensations you are experiencing. That's all. Feel the contact between your body and the ground beneath it. Feel the weight of your body and relax into the unconditional support of the ground.

- Then begin scanning your awareness from the tips of your toes to the crown of your head (a full-body scan), relaxing as you go. Take at least 10 minutes for this if you can, or continue until your entire body has relaxed into awareness.

- Now, simply rest. Don't do anything. Drop any idea of trying to do anything. Just rest. Rest in the moment. Be aware of whatever comes to you. If you feel yourself starting to slip into sleep, bring your attention back to the flow of your breath, the sounds in the room and your contact with the surface beneath you. If you feel that you are about to black out, you might like to lightly contract your fingers or toes as a way of bringing yourself back to bodily awareness.

- Allow yourself to rest in this mindful awareness of the hypnagogic state for the rest of your session. When your mind drifts off, use awareness of your breath or the hypnagogic imagery to bring yourself back to the present moment.

- Either end your practice when your alarm goes off or allow yourself to slip into sleep if you are using this practice as a precursor to sleep.

....

Charlie says

'I have a 25-minute guided audio-track version of this practice called "The Tao of Dozing", taken from an album of guided meditations called Lucid Dreaming, Conscious Sleeping. *It's available on the* Empower You Unlimited Audio *app, or from wherever you purchase your audiobooks.'*

Hypnagogic Creativity

The hypnagogic state is a wonderfully creative place in which intuitive ideas flow effortlessly as our brain switches from the linear, logical, left-brain dominance of the day to the intuitive, imaginative, right-brain dominance of the night. Although hypnagogic imagery may seem to be nothing more than the unintelligible side-effect of the brain 'shutting down' ready for sleep, it's actually much more than this.

For hundreds of years, both left- and right-brainers have been using the hypnagogic state as a kind of 'holodeck' for creative problem-solving and thinking outside the box of logical thought. Its unique combination of right-brain dominance and wakeful awareness makes it the perfect place to see ideas in a new light.

Edison, the inventor of the light bulb, used to engage the hypnagogic state for creative problem-solving, and even accredited his final design for the light bulb to a revelation that he had while drifting into a hypnagogic nap.

Each afternoon, he would prepare an armchair with two metal plates on the floor under the armrests. He would then hold ball bearings in his hands, place them on the armrests and have a nap.[4] As he dozed, the ideas and research that he had been working on would float into his mind and stew in the creative juices of the hypnagogic state. When his body entered full sleep, muscle paralysis would set in and the ball bearings in his hands would be released, hit the metal plates below and wake him up, allowing him to jot down any new revelations or ideas.

Salvador Dali was also partial to a bit of hypnagogic roving and would often use his hypnagogia as inspiration for his work, which, when combined with a pint of absinthe, presumably led to the 100-foot elephants stepping over melting clocks.

Dali had a slightly different technique, though. He would lie down on a couch and put a champagne glass on the floor. He would then carefully place one end of a spoon on the edge of the glass and the other end in his hand. He would float into the hypnagogic state, mindful of all the imagery, and when his hypnagogic state became full REM dreaming and muscle paralysis set in, he would naturally lose his grip on the spoon, which would crash into the glass noisily enough to wake him. He would then immediately sketch the bizarre hypnagogic imagery that he had witnessed.[5]

More recently, a 2001 Harvard study found proof that the hypnagogic state really was a great place for creative problem-solving. The researchers concluded that although full-blown dreams were great for working with and reflecting upon psychological issues, the hypnagogic state was especially effective at 'problem solving that benefited from hallucinatory images being critically examined while still before the eyes'.[6] This is because hypnagogic imagery can be evaluated consciously as it manifests and so it becomes a much more accessible source of creativity than full-blown dreams, which have to be remembered and interpreted before their meaning is revealed.

Hypnopompic Mindfulness (Snooze Button Meditation)

The hypnopompic state is as creative and imaginative a state as the hypnagogic, but because it occurs after the psychological processing of sleep and dreaming, it contains a clarity and vastness unmatched by the hypnagogic. Whereas the hypnagogic is characterized by imagery and visuals, the hypnopompic is often more of a blank canvas, a clear, non-conceptual awareness dawning like the day. By accessing the hypnopompic, we are gaining insight into our mind at its clearest and most radiant, with the clutter of daytime residues and chattering thoughts filed away. For many people, mindfulness meditation applied in the hypnopompic can be one of the most refined experiences of pure consciousness that they have.

Rob Nairn was a hypnopompic specialist and it was his idea to introduce the practice of hypnopompic mindfulness into the retreats and workshops that we ran. Rob actually believed that this practice offered the potential 'for a level of profound psychological exploration unmatched by any other state of mind'.[7] He also thought that it might be even more beneficial than lucid dreaming, because although it can take a while to get to grips with lucid dreaming, you can learn hypnopompic mindfulness within a couple of sessions.

The hypnopompic state dawns like a vast expanse of stillness and calm after our often emotionally charged dreams, and if we can learn to rest within it, we will often gain insight into the nature and meaning of the dreams we have just been having with far greater ease than if we reflect upon them once fully awake.*

In a nutshell, if you want to tap into your full psychological potential, hit the snooze button.

---

* Ayang Rinpoche says that during sleep the energy of our consciousness collects at the heart centre, where the mind is said to reside. This means that our first thought is particularly important, because it infuses the whole mind with its flavour, so try to think a loving, joyful thought on waking.

....

Let's Snooze!

• The hypnopompic state can only be entered from full sleep. If you can, try to enter it naturally by allowing yourself to wake up slowly and mindfully in the morning, without opening your eyes if possible. Simply become mindful of that brief space between sleep and wakefulness that you pass through every time you wake up.

• When you feel yourself partially waking up and entering this state, don't open your eyes, don't move your body and try not to engage too much 'thinking' as such – just lie there mindfully aware. The hypnopompic is a vast space in which awareness can naturally rest, so do just that, while remaining mindful of any spontaneous insights that might arise.

• For many of us, entering the hypnopompic naturally can be a bit tricky, due to our habitual use of an alarm clock, but not to worry. If you can't enter it naturally, just set your alarm 10 or 20 minutes before you intend to wake up. Make sure that the alarm is within easy reach, and when it sounds, wake up very gently (without opening your eyes if possible) and hit the 10- or 20-minute snooze button mindfully, in a calm, unhurried way.*

• After you've hit the snooze button, close your eyes (if you needed to open them) and become aware of your breathing. Due to the nature of the hypnopompic, a simple awareness of breath meditation is all that's needed here: simply knowing when you're breathing in and when you're breathing out.

• If you feel yourself slipping back into sleep, just bring yourself back to the awareness of your breath and the feeling of your body being supported by the bed.

---

* On the retreats I run, I use the high-pitched tone of a singing bowl to bring people out of sleep and into the hypnopompic state, but you can use any sound that rouses you out of sleep.

- Allow your mind to rest in the broad panoramic warmth of the hypnopompic state. After 10 or 20 minutes, the snooze alarm will sound again, which is when you can either wake up fully or repeat the exercise.

Charlie says

'The hypnopompic often gets overlooked because it's mistakenly seen as the mind at its bleariest, but this is often just because we haven't had enough sleep. If we can enter the hypnopompic refreshed and are able to maintain awareness within it, morning grogginess will be a thing of the past and we'll be able to start every morning mindfully aware.'

It should be noted that the enhanced clarity of the hypnopompic also means a lack of self-censorship, which often shines a light into the dark corners of our mind and sometimes reveals our deepest fears and neuroses, which we unconsciously repress during our waking hours. But if we can learn to rest in this state with non-judgemental awareness, simply witnessing, we will naturally begin to integrate these neuroses into the wholeness of ourselves. As the great Krishnamurti once said, 'The seeing is the doing.'[8]

People who struggle with sleep often spend a lot of time in the hypnopompic in the middle of the night, as they wake up after a few hours of slumber and then can't get back to sleep. This is a state often referred to as 'the 4 a.m. demons', as the clarity of the hypnopompic can often highlight the current preoccupations of the mind.

This state can actually be a beacon of light in a night of sleeplessness, but most people reject it, fearing it out of habit, whereas in fact it is part of the wonderfully beneficial hour of the wolf...

The Hour of the Wolf

It's 4 a.m. and you're wide awake. It seems as though everybody else in the whole world is asleep and you're awake. You're abnormal. You're a freak.

No, you're not a freak – you're a wolf.

The hour of the wolf is what millions of people could appreciate and experience with fascination if they could only drop the expectation that they should be asleep during it. In fact, I am writing this paragraph at 4.10 a.m., feeling full of ideas and inspiration.

Jeff Warren, author of *The Head Trip*, the wonderfully researched travelogue of the human mind, believes that waking at this time of night, which he calls 'the Watch', is actually a very natural phenomenon that harks back to our pre-industrial sleep cycle. Yes, before the industrial revolution of the 1800s – and thus for a much longer period of human history – people slept very differently. Most people in northern Europe and Britain, plus many in countries under the control of the British Empire, slept in two bouts: from about 9 p.m. to midnight (allowing for seasonal fluctuations) and from about 2 a.m. to dawn.

So, what happened between midnight and 2 a.m? People were doing stuff! They might go and check on their cows in the fields, or they might go to a friend's place and have a drink, or they might have sex, but whatever they chose to do, they would be wide awake.

In all probability, we slept in that way for thousands of years and many populations untouched by Western industrialization still have a similar sleeping pattern today. With anthropological research finding more than 500 other cross-cultural references to this distinct 'two sleeps' pattern,[9] it can be assumed to have been an almost-universal norm.

So it seems that 'human beings have been hardwired from prehistoric times to spend a good portion of their nocturnal hours in a resting state that lies somewhere between wakefulness and sleep.'[10]

But one question remains: what happened to change that sleeping pattern?

The industrial revolution happened. Warren tells us that three developments that accompanied it soon came to affect the sleeping patterns of Londoners, and with London being the centre of the industrialized world, the sleeping patterns of much of humanity. Coffee, affordable books and, crucially, artificial lighting were, along with the factory owners' desire to work their employees for longer hours, three of the contributing factors that changed the way we slept, because people could stay awake longer, tanked up on caffeine, reading affordable novels by (eventually) the light of an Edison electric bulb.

Who would have thought that three seemingly unrelated developments could combine to affect our lives so dramatically, without us even realizing it?

Charlie says

'If you are someone who wakes in the middle of the night and feels unable to go back to sleep, don't fret – you might be displaying a much more natural sleeping pattern than the rest of us. Perhaps people who swear that they feel fine after four or five hours of sleep really do feel fine, but, regrettably, they aren't allowing themselves the second bout of sleep that is waiting for them in the wings.'

Nobody sleeps for eight solid hours, however much it may seem that way. Sleep is a constant state of flux, moving tidally throughout the night, coursing from the shallows to the depths. David Neubauer, author of *Understanding Sleeplessness*, says: 'Thinking it's necessary to stay asleep for eight hours straight may be unrealistic… but since we're conditioned to think that waking during the night is a problem, when it happens, we panic, a reaction that causes our brains to awaken even further.'[11]

Multiple wake-ups throughout the night are fine, too, and even waking every 90 minutes or so can be part of a healthy sleep pattern. We tend to sleep in roughly 90-minute cycles, so brief awakenings after each cycle are natural and don't affect our sleep detrimentally.

Most of us do have brief awakenings throughout the night, but we ordinarily don't have any memory of them. Those struggling with sleep, however, because of their hyperconscious fear of not being able to sleep when they 'should' be asleep, tend to grasp at these micro-awakenings to fuel the negative expectation that they should be asleep, and so perpetuate the cycle.

If you do find that you wake up in the early hours and can't get back to sleep, try to drop the expectation of sleeping and definitely don't try to fall asleep.* Instead, either practise hypnopompic mindfulness (especially if you class yourself as an insomniac) or simply enjoy the cortically rich, alert clarity of the hour of the wolf and use it creatively, as I am doing right now as I type this paragraph into my phone.

Napping

When I was in my early twenties, I hardly ever took naps. I was far too busy trying to change the world. But now I realize that if you really want to change the world, you should take a nap.

A nap – any short period of sleep outside your main sleep cycle – is one of the most beneficial things that you can do for both your psychological and physiological health. Napping charges your body with potential, and whatever activities you engage in after a nap will be executed more easily and tackled more creatively.[12]

---

* Rob Nairn once told me, 'Insomnia is the process of *trying* to fall asleep.'

A 2009 Harvard University study has shown that those who nap regularly are 37 per cent less likely to die of heart disease than non-nappers, with male nappers reducing their chance of heart disease even more, by up to 64 per cent.[13] There is no daily medicine that can reduce a man's chances of dying from heart disease by that much, so naps do offer really quite incredible results. Heart disease is one of the biggest killers in the Western world and if medical science produced a new pill that could reduce men's risk of dying from it by 64 per cent, they'd all be queuing up to buy it. There's no need to queue: just have a snooze.

As well as being great for the body and mind, napping is also great for lucid dreaming. During an afternoon nap, we tend to enter light sleep and then REM much more quickly and to stay there for most of the nap without much entry into delta-wave deep sleep, if any at all. This allows you to have lucid dreams during the daytime too.

Chinese Taoist dream yogis saw from early on that having only one opportunity per day to enter the dream state wasn't enough for serious dream yoga practice and so they made daily napping a central part of their tradition. They realized that by napping during the day we would enter our full sleep cycle at night with our body already quite rested, so sleep wouldn't be engaged in out of fatigue but more deliberately for the goal of spiritual practice.

Naps provide great neurological benefits for the lucid dreamer, too. Biological psychologists have discovered that 'habitual nappers' have greater alpha and theta EEG power in stages one and two of sleep,[14] meaning that their brain capacity is actually enhanced throughout REM sleep, thus aiding lucidity. Suddenly an afternoon nap doesn't seem so lazy, after all.

Feel free to nap whenever you want, but make sure that it ends at least six hours before you intend to go to bed. This is in order to give your body enough time to build up its 'sleep pressure', the biological basis of tiredness.

And try not to nap for more than 60–90 minutes, because anything over that may lead you into delta-wave sleep, which might make you feel a bit groggy when you wake up from it. Most people find that a nap of between 20 and 60 minutes is best.

And if you can't nap, then at least rest. Whether it's termed a 'controlled recovery period' (CRP) or 'non-sleep deep rest' (NSDR) or Yoga Nidra, there is growing body of evidence to show that simply resting deeply for half an hour a day does wonders for mental health.

This could be as much as a full-on 60-minute Yoga Nidra session or as little as a 30-minute eyes-closed rest in a darkened room, or anything in between. The point is to allow your body to do nothing other than rest, recover and relax for at least 30 minutes a day.

Charlie says

'I was in a lucid dream once when I invoked the presence of the Tibetan master Guru Padmasambhava. When he appeared, I asked him, "How can I be of most benefit to all beings?", to which he replied, "Take a nap." I guess I was expecting something a bit more profound, but I've taken his advice to heart nonetheless!'

Creating a Practice

'For the first time in my life I was looking forward to going to sleep....'[15]
Carlos Castaneda

So, you now have a fully stocked toolbox of daytime, night-time and liminal state techniques.

There is a Zen Buddhist teaching that says spiritual practice is like eating food: you can't gain the nourishment of food just from reading about it, talking about it or learning about the ingredients – you actually have to eat it. It's exactly the same with lucid dreaming.

You might already be applying all the techniques and having lucid dreams, or you may still be working on your dream recall. Either is totally fine. Work at the pace best suited to you.

And feel free to use whatever combination of techniques works well for you, but here is a step-by-step protocol that I recommend as a starting-point for beginner dream yogis.

Step by Step

The first thing to do is to create a dream plan. It has to excite you and it has to be worth the effort. A boring dream plan will lead to a slow and fruitless practice, so aim big: meet God, heal a chronic illness, experience enlightenment. Whatever it is, make sure it makes you salivate!

You are going to have multiple lucid dreams and so you'll make and complete multiple dream plans as you progress, but focus on one dream plan at a time.

Once you've made your dream plan, you might want to spend at least the next week or so just concentrating on your dream recall and documenting your dreams, so that you have a really firm basis for your practice. Aim to be recalling at least one dream a night if you can.

Solid dream recall also means solid dream sign recognition, because the more dreams you recall, the more dream signs you'll notice. Once you start to become aware of your dream signs, you'll start to become aware of them while you are dreaming, which may well lead to your first lucid dream.

Spend the next week or so really focusing on recognizing your dream signs. This is where reality checks come in, as sometimes even though we recognize a dream sign, the rest of the dream looks so realistic that we just can't believe that we're actually dreaming. That's exactly the situation in which to perform a reality check.

How will you actually remember to do reality checks in your dreams? By getting into the habit of doing them while you're awake: the Weird Technique. You can either start doing this straight away or after a week or two of focusing mainly on dream recall and dream signs. Add to all this the night-time practices of Hypnagogic Affirmation, FAC, MILD and the rest and you'll have a pretty solid lucid dreaming protocol to follow.

And make sure you're getting enough sleep. The probability of having a lucid dream in the last two hours of sleep is more than twice as great as in the previous hours of sleep. This means that you can almost double your chances of having a lucid dream by extending your sleep by an extra two hours.* Still try to wake briefly at your normal time, though, rather than just sleeping straight through for the extra two hours, because then you get a chance to drop back into sleep while practising a lucidity technique.

Interestingly, from the perspective of Tibetan medicine, which sees our sleep cycle as broken up into stages of influence from each of the three humours of the body (bile, phlegm and subtle wind energy), the last two hours of the sleep cycle, based on an average eight-hour cycle, is when we experience 'the most balanced state of subtle wind energy' and is thus the best time to engage in dream yoga practice.

The main things that support a lucid dreaming practice are enthusiasm and determination, though, so focus on those by asking yourself, 'Why do I want to lucid dream?' and 'Am I actually determined to do the practice rather than just think or read about it?'

---

* If you already get seven or eight hours of sleep, then you can take that up to 10 hours, but no more. Regularly having over 10 hours of sleep has been shown to be detrimental to health.

Some of you will get lucid tonight simply from the enthused determination to do so, whereas others will take a couple of weeks to have their first lucid dream. At an in-person weekend workshop I will teach all the lucid dreaming techniques described previously in just two days, whereas on an online course I will spread them out over six weeks, so feel free to set your own schedule and take it at your own pace.

Charlie says

'If you want to go deeper into lucid dreaming, please do check out all my courses and workshops at www.charliemorley.com. You can join me online or in person at a lucid dreaming retreat, and I have monthly online drop-in sessions too, which are free and open to all.'

Be a Salmon

And my final piece of advice for creating a lucid dreaming practice is to take inspiration from the humble salmon.

Most fish tend to go with the flow and swim downstream, but not the salmon. The salmon swims upstream. Why? To return to the place where it was born and to spawn new life there.

One day something awakens within the salmon: a yearning to return home. And so it makes a choice – a choice to do things differently, a choice to stand out from the shoal. It decides to swim upstream to find its way home.

The salmon's journey up the river isn't random. It has a form of inbuilt GPS that allows it to use the magnetic field of the Earth to find the exact bend on the exact part of the exact river where it was born. Its journey home is encoded in its DNA.

As the salmon swims upstream, passing all the fish who are swimming the other way, I can imagine them laughing at it and saying, 'Hey, you're crazy! Why don't you just go with the flow?'

And I can imagine that for a minute the salmon might question itself and think, *Why am I doing this? Why don't I just go with the flow like everybody else?*

And then it remembers, *I'm making my way home.* And so it ignores the other fish, it's proud of its different path and it continues on the road less travelled, or swum.

The Buddha described the spiritual path as 'going against the stream'. He believed that although the way that everyone else was going might be the easy way, it wasn't the way to freedom, it wasn't the way home.

To step onto the spiritual path (and definitely onto the path of lucid dreaming) is to be like a salmon and to allow that encoding in our DNA to take us back to the place of creation.

So I urge you not to just 'go with the flow' of the masses who think that 'work, eat, sleep, repeat' is all that life can be. Be like a salmon.

Don't disregard your dreams and see sleep as wasted time. Be like a salmon.

And when others question you, saying, 'What good is lucid dreaming anyway?', shout back joyfully, 'I am finding my way back home! Wake up, come join me and be like a salmon!'

Of course, like a salmon, you'll encounter obstacles on your journey and in Part III we'll learn how to embrace them...

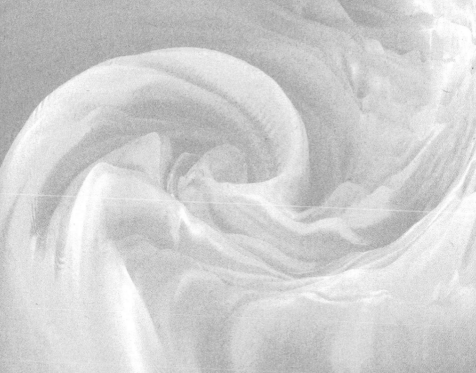

PART III

GERMINATION

CHAPTER 10

EMBRACING THE OBSTACLES OF THE NIGHT

'If you can find a path with no obstacles,
it probably doesn't lead anywhere.'

Frank A. Clark

Now that we have prepared the ground and set out on the path, we can move into the Germination process. Here we'll explore out-of-body experiences, prophetic dreams, experiencing Oneness, and how lucid dreaming is one of the most powerful treatments for post-traumatic stress currently available.

But before all that, let's look at the obstacles we might meet.

As our seeds of lucidity start to sprout, they may encounter rocks and weeds as they follow the sunlight to the surface. This is totally natural, and in fact some of the rocks might provide solid foundations for roots to form around. Let's explore some of the obstacles that we might encounter.

Many may seem detrimental to our dream practice – everything from recurring nightmares to missing a night's sleep altogether – but I've found that most of these obstacles can be skilfully embraced, and some are more like dragons guarding pots of gold and the treasures of lucidity. So, let's meet our dragons...

Performance Anxiety

Lucid dreaming may not be particularly easy to master, but in all the years that I've taught it, I've yet to encounter a person who cannot learn how to do it.

Sometimes, though, we do all the prep, set all the alarms, do everything right and then... nothing happens.

I've taught people who've had their first-ever lucid dream after a 30-minute drop-in workshop at a music festival, but I've also taught people who've done eight-week courses and weekend retreats, read all the books on the subject and still struggled to get lucid regularly.

We're all working from wonderfully different starting-points of mental capacity, dream recall and motivation, and this leads to a plethora of different successes and challenges along the path of lucid dreaming. Nevertheless, I can say with certainty that if you apply sustained effort with strong motivation, your first lucid dream will definitely come, and once you have tasted lucidity for the first time, it will be much easier to taste it again.

'The chains of habit are often too weak to be felt until they are too strong to be broken',[1] so don't feel discouraged if it seems that you're making slow progress, because you may be just one more night away from your tipping point, a breakthrough moment that will make all the hard work seem worth its weight in gold. Lucidity training is cumulative, and each night of training (regardless of whether you become lucid or not) fills up your lucidity tank, drop by drop. You might be just one drop away from a lucid dream.

One of the major problems with lucid dream practice is the name 'lucid dreaming'. The aim is in the name, which leads people to think that they are outright failures if they don't achieve this aim. Let me clarify... In the game of baseball, the aim is to score home runs, but the name of the game isn't 'home run ball', it's baseball. Why? Because baseball is about proceeding through the bases, not just about hitting the home runs. It's the same with lucid dreaming. Just as you can be a great baseball player without having hit many home runs, so you can be a great lucid dreamer without having had many lucid dreams. Remember, just one lucid dream can change your life forever.

If you aren't having any lucid dreams yet, you might be a great hypnopompic mindfulness meditator, or have great dream recall, or experience powerful shadow integration in your non-lucid dreams. All these are great attributes to have on the playing field of lucidity, yet none of them are determined by having a lucid dream.

Fifteen years ago, a lady on my first-ever course told me, 'I haven't even had my first lucid dream yet, but I can say for sure that the act of sleeping will never be the same again. I can't unknow what I've learned about the sleep stages, the process of dreaming, the hypnagogic states… Falling asleep will never be the same again.'

The experience of that student was actually more important to me than the experiences of all the students who were lucid from week one, because what it showed me was that the process of learning how to bring awareness into sleep and dreaming had profoundly changed a lifetime of habitual tendency.

There have been times when I've had four of five fully lucid dreams in one night, but often I will go weeks without any lucidity and feel a total fraud. I lose my confidence and start to doubt myself. Because I doubt myself, I stop training. Because I stop training, my lucidity tank runs dry. And finally I feel that I've lost my ability forever, I'll be forced to quit teaching, my books will be burned and catastrophe is looming! Such drama.

How do I get myself back on track when I fall into this kind of melodramatic ego trap? I relax, I stop trying and I make friends with my feelings of failure. I rekindle my inspiration by reading a new book on the subject or watching a dream-themed film, and most importantly, I talk to someone. I open up about my fears, doubts and feelings of failure, knowing that this will free them and allow my lucid awareness to flow back to me naturally. It always does.

Those of you who haven't had a lucid dream yet may think, *I don't have any ability!*, but remember that you used to lucid dream all time when you were a child... And even if you haven't had a lucid dream yet as an adult, I'm sure that you've had some success in being aware of the hypnagogic and hypnopompic states or recalling your dreams. In fact, just by reading this book you're creating the causes and conditions that will lead to lucidity.

You can feel confident that lucidity will come soon as long as you keep practising. I've come across many people who have got lucid on their first night of practice and others who have taken six months to have their first lucid dream. True confidence comes from the knowledge that you've put in the hard work, and confidence based on this knowledge is like the varnish on the treasure chest, sealing the grain of the wood, preserving and protecting its lustre. So, have confidence in yourself – you are a lucid dreamer!

The American philosopher Ralph Waldo Emerson said, 'Enthusiasm is the mother of effort – without it, nothing great was ever achieved.' If you want to learn how to lucid dream regularly, then lucid dreaming has to be something you're enthusiastic about. Lama Zangmo, the female lama who runs the Buddhist centre where I used to live, says that the most important aspect of lucid dream training is enthusiasm. She told me, 'The main thing is to have a very strong intention. You have to be fired up for it, you have to really want to do it!'[2]

Charlie says

'Dreams occur in the mind, so they are directly influenced by your state of mind. If you go to sleep doubting your ability to have lucid dreams or not trusting in the techniques, then this will naturally hinder your ability to get lucid. Go to sleep in a joyful, confident state of mind and I'm confident that the techniques will work for you.'

The most important thing to remember is this: don't just fall asleep. Try to do something, however small, each and every night. If you're struggling with lucidity, train in your daytime reality checks. If you're struggling with dream recall, work on your daily mindfulness. If you're too tired at night to stay awake, take a nap during the day. There are so many ways in which you can engage this practice, so don't put it off, do something today. Make a change, however small. In the words of the poet John Greenleaf Whittier, 'For all the sad words of tongue or pen, the saddest are these: it might have been.'[3]

Nightmares

Many people view nightmares as one of the biggest obstacles to sleep and dreaming practice, because they create fear around the process of dreaming, which makes us not want to go to sleep in the first place.

Nightmares occur in REM sleep. They can occur for a variety of reasons, such as mental and physical illness (and often as a side-effect of the drugs used to treat that illness), as a result of post-traumatic stress or sometimes just as expressions of a mind trying to prepare itself for possible future threat.

Sometimes a nightmare is a straight replay of a traumatic experience, but often the traumatized part of ourselves takes on a more symbolic form. For example, if a person is in an abusive relationship, although they may well have nightmares in which the abuser appears, often the nightmares are symbolic – for example, being in a flooded room with the water level rising dangerously – because that's what the abuse or coercive control feels like.

Whether a nightmare is a straight replay of trauma or symbolic, one of the unique aspects of lucid dreaming is the ability to communicate directly with these manifestations of mind. So, however a nightmare manifests, rather than running from it, fighting it or rejecting it, if we can become lucid, we can embrace it with the compassionate realization that it is merely a mental representation of our own trauma, which we now have the valuable opportunity to integrate.

For lucid dreamers, nightmares are opportunities. They can be embraced, transformed and used as mediums of getting lucid. The first time I went on retreat with Rob Nairn, somebody asked him at breakfast how he had slept, to which he replied, 'Very well! I had some wonderful nightmares!' At the time I thought he was mad, but years later I discovered what he meant, because for lucid dreamers, nightmares are such good news.

At a meeting of the European Science Foundation in 2009 it was suggested that lucid dreaming was such an effective remedy for curing chronic nightmares that it could be offered as a mainstream treatment,[4] and a 2013 neurobiological study from Brazil concluded that lucid dreaming could be used 'as a therapy for recurrent nightmares, a common symptom of post-traumatic stress disorder'.[5]

Most of the time, nightmares are good for us and are actually supportive of our mental health. They help us heal, they draw our attention to emotional wounds that we may be blindsided by while awake and they update our evolutionary survival mechanisms.

I've written about nightmares extensively in both *Dreaming Through Darkness* and my 2022 book about trauma-affected sleep, *Wake Up to Sleep*, so check out those books if you want to go deeper. But for now, let's at least touch on what I call the 'Three

Reframes', because they may just change the way you look at nightmares forever.

A Dream That Is Shouting

A nightmare is simply a dream that is shouting. It is shouting, 'Hey, look at this! Deal with this fear!' or 'Over here! This trauma needs attention!'

Just as physical pain is used by our brain to draw our attention to a wounded part of our body, so nightmares are used by our unconscious mind to draw our attention to a wounded part of our psyche. The nightmare isn't shouting in order to scare us, but to help us. And so, if we want to integrate our nightmares, we need to do everything we can to tell our unconscious mind, 'OK, OK! I'm listening!' How? By writing our nightmares down, by talking about them, drawing them or doing whatever else we can to show that we're listening.

A Sign of a Healing Mind

If we cut our arm, it bleeds, and then white blood cells coagulate to form a scab over the cut. This allows the healing process to continue below the surface. If this didn't happen, we might end up with sepsis or gangrene from every minor wound. A nightmare works in a similar way to a scab: it's a manifestation of the healing process that creates a protective layer over the wound to allow healing to occur beneath the surface. Just like a scab, it can be itchy and unsightly and we might try to hide it from others, and yet it's vital to the healing process.

One study from Rush University in Chicago showed that in many cases healing was actually predicated on 'dreaming about the emotional themes and sentiments of the waking state trauma'[6] and that 'only patients who were expressly dreaming about the painful experiences' around the time of them actually happening became clinically free of their depression.

> **Charlie says**
>
> *'Of course, I'm not suggesting that we have to have nightmares in order to heal, but if trauma remains unwitnessed and thus unintegrated, our mind's natural self-healing mechanism will often use nightmares as its preferred means of integration.'*

An Evolutionary Tool

Nightmares may be part of what makes us human. Antti Revonsuo, a Finnish scientist who 'collects nightmares', believes that they are rehearsals for the daily struggle to survive. He says, 'Nightmares force us to go through simulated threatening events in order that in the waking world we are more prepared to survive them because we have been training for them in our dreams.'[7] He goes on to say that the reason children frequently have nightmares about wild animals, even if they live in urban areas devoid of such threats, is an inheritance from early humans, who would be faced with life-threatening wild beasts on a daily basis, and that in fact this proves just how vital nightmares were to the evolution of our species. He even speculates, 'Without nightmares, there is a good chance that humanity would not exist.'[8]

There is also a good chance that lucid dreaming wouldn't exist either, because so many lucid dreams begin as nightmares or anxiety dreams. This shows that nightmares are a blessing in disguise and really are the dragons guarding the gold.

To understand the reason for nightmarish fear preceding lucid dreams so frequently, we first need to understand the reason for fear in the waking state. The biological purpose of fear is to make us scan our surroundings more carefully and so become more aware of a potential threat or danger. Fear maximizes blood flow to the major muscle groups and to the brain, which increases our sensory perception, allowing us to deal with the potential threat with a heightened level of awareness. Heightened awareness? Maximized blood flow to the brain? Increase of sensory perception? No wonder nightmares lead to lucidity! So much of what we need to get lucid is produced as a side-effect of fear, so when we experience a fearful nightmare, our awareness is often boosted into lucidity.

Fear within dreams can also help us spot dream signs. In 2009, research at the Erasmus University in Rotterdam found that the experience of fear 'enhances our ability to identify coarse-grain features in preference to fine details'.[9] Of course, if we're being attacked, we don't care if our attacker has wrinkles, we just care about how threatening their movements are. If we apply this to dreaming, we can see that when we experience fear in the dream state, our attention will be drawn away from the often deceptively convincing detail of the dreamscape and into a wider visual perspective, which may help us to recognize a previously unnoticed dream sign.

And, as we learned before, from a Buddhist point of view, nightmares can be a great training ground for fearlessness. In fact, the great Tibetan lama Tsongkhapa commented way back in the 15th century that nightmares were the easiest way to get lucid.

Fear is one of the greatest obstacles on the spiritual path and can often form the basis of major psychological blocks. In the after-death *bardo* state, fear is said to be our biggest obstacle, because the *bardo* journey is so intense that for many of us it is an experience of terror, shock and awe. But if we can train in fearlessness through lucid nightmares and create a habit of calm awareness in preference to fear and panic, this will be a huge benefit to us in the after-death *bardo* state.

Quite simply, nightmares can be a blessing for the lucid dreamer and lucid dreaming is a blessing for those who suffer from nightmares.

Night Terrors

A night terror is quite different from a nightmare. Whereas nightmares usually occur in REM sleep, night terrors are typically associated with non-dreaming sleep and are 'pure emotional experiences that occur upon awakening from sleep',[10] so they aren't actually linked with dreaming at all. They are episodes of extreme panic and fear that occur in the transition from deep sleep to the hypnopompic state, experiences of unadulterated terror, a bit like a night-time panic attack. Subjects may sit bolt upright in bed with their eyes open, screaming, and be unable to be roused from this state for several minutes. Those most frequently affected are children aged between three and 12 years old and adults working with PTSD.

The saving grace of night terrors is that the sufferer often has no memory of them, and due to the fact that their mind is in the relaxed state of slow-wave sleep, the renowned sleep researcher William Dement believes they may not be experiencing fear at all, because it is their body that is expressing fright rather than their mind.

Charlie says

'It's young children who most often experience night terrors, and although this usually freaks their parents out, it's not usually a cause for concern. It's thought that night terrors may be caused by the nervous system still maturing and so they often pass as the child grows up.'

Sleep Paralysis

From the Japanese *kanashibari*, 'fastened in metal', to the African 'witch riding your back' to incubus/succubus myths of the West, the phenomenon of the brain waking up from sleep but the body staying paralysed has been mythologized in almost every culture. Thankfully, we now have a neurological explanation for sleep paralysis, which helps to put the demonic myths of the past to bed.

Sleep paralysis is caused by one of the three REM sleep systems (muscular paralysis), staying engaged when the other two (sensory blockade and cortical activation) have been disengaged, meaning that while your brain has partially woken up and your senses are taking in partial sensory input, your physical body cannot move.

Sleep paralysis most commonly occurs during the hypnopompic state, but sometimes in the hypnagogic, too, and is an often hallucinatory experience in which the subject may feel totally awake and the room that they wake up in may look exactly the same as it normally does, but due to the brain's momentary engagement in both the dream state and waking state, there may be hallucinatory images superimposed over the normal field of vision, and often loud audio hallucinations, too.

This can be a terrifying experience, but it is a terror that is mostly rooted in the mystery of the situation. Waking up and feeling that your body is paralysed leads to intense fear, which can also lead to hyperventilation, which, when combined with the bodily paralysis, can lead to a feeling of pressure or weight on your chest. This often goes together with hypnagogic hallucinations, which are aural and visual dream aspects superimposed on the waking world and reflective of your terrified mental state. Now add to the mix the fact that sleep paralysis is often accompanied by a form of hyperacusis (a condition in which sounds become amplified and distorted) and we can see why in earlier times possession by a demon often seemed the best explanation for such experiences.*

---

* Some researchers believe that alien abductions can often be put down to misinterpreted sleep paralysis. If you look at the timings and the actual subjective reports, the argument does seem to hold some weight, but as a workshop participant once countered, maybe the aliens are just waiting for us to get sleep paralysis before they abduct us!

Charlie says

'I woke up in my bed and looked around the room. I was unable to move and there was a dark ominous presence around me. There was a pressure on my chest. I felt a scaly hand cover my face. It had claws. I could feel them across my cheekbones. I began to panic. Someone was in my room. Alien life forms were about to abduct me! Then suddenly it hit me: Hang on, this is sleep paralysis! It's all a hallucination! This is so cool!'

If you want to break free from sleep paralysis while you're experiencing it, the best course of action is to relax and exhale (or imagine exhaling) one long breath through your front teeth, making a sound similar to letting air out of a tyre. This relaxation of the respiratory system will help to disengage the paralysis mechanism and bring you back into your rational mind. Think of yourself as a diver who knows that they must come up to the surface slowly and without panic if they are to avoid the bends. Just relax, breathe out and follow the bubbles to the surface.

Although sleep paralysis may seem to go on for hours, it rarely lasts for more than a couple of minutes and is quite a common occurrence. It isn't anything to be feared or dreaded. Most probably you haven't been possessed by demons, you aren't going mad and there aren't any dark forces in your bedroom. You are safe, and all that is happening is that your brain has woken up before your body has.

Those training in lucid dreaming should be grateful for sleep paralysis, because during it you have one foot in the dream world and one in the waking world – the perfect state from which to drop into a lucid dream.*

---

* Sleep paralysis can become quite common among people who are learning to dream lucidly (due to the increased awareness of the hypnopompic they develop) and is often actually a sign of progression along the path.

False Awakenings

'All that we see, or seem to see,
is but a dream within a dream.'
Edgar Allan Poe

Charlie says

'I woke up in my bed and reached for the bedside lamp. I flicked the switch, but it wouldn't turn on. The bulb had blown. I sat up, unplugged the lamp and unscrewed the bulb. I shook it and heard the rattle of the blown filament. I looked closely and could see the fragments of the blown filament inside the glass bulb. I reached over to replace the bulb and suddenly remembered that I don't even have a bedside lamp. No way! *I thought. Then I woke up in my bed – for real this time.'*

Welcome to the weird world of false awakenings...

A false awakening is the experience of dreaming that we've woken up when we are in fact still dreaming. We might dream that we've woken up in our bed as normal, with our bedroom looking identical to real life, until suddenly we wake up from this dream within a dream to actual waking reality. Some people even have multiple false awakenings in which they dream of waking up, getting out of bed and then waking up again. So they get out of bed again, reflect on their previous false awakening and then suddenly they wake up again, for real this time: a dream within a dream within a dream.

Although they sometimes happen spontaneously, false awakenings often manifest when people start doing lucid dream training because they set such a strong intent to 'wake up in their dreams' that they dream about waking up. They are very strange experiences and have been described by some researchers as 'a lucid dream – minus the lucidity'.[11]

191

The 'reality' of a false awakening often seems absolutely identical to waking reality, including a perfectly detailed carbon copy of our bedroom without any aspect seeming dreamlike at all, but if we get into the habit of doing a reality check as soon as we wake up (or think we wake up), we can transform every false awakening we have into a lucid dream.

Becoming lucid within a false awakening can be one the most bizarre experiences in the lucid dream canon, because the reality that we find ourselves in is so utterly undreamlike – often a direct carbon copy of our bedroom, a mentally constructed *doppelgänger* of reality – that it calls into question the very nature of the waking state.

In late 2010, as part of my research for this section of the book, I set out to intentionally have as many false awakenings as I could. I managed to have seven fully lucid false awakenings in a row or a 'dream within a dream within a dream within a dream...' – you get the idea. The first false awakening was quite dreamy, and I could fly about and affect the dream easily through mental intent, but each subsequent awakening brought with it a decrease in volitional influence and an increase in the 'normality' of the dreamscape.

By the sixth false awakening, hand reality checks were barely working, I was unable to fly and my ability to transform the dreamscape was very weak. With each successive false awakening, I seemed to be coming closer and closer to waking reality. This made me wonder if our waking reality was the final level of wakefulness or just another false awakening in which we were yet to get lucid. With spiritual realization being so often referred to as 'awakening from a dream', perhaps this isn't such a crazy proposition. Who knows?

And now let's explore one obstacle that blights the lives of so many and yet can be treated so effectively through lucid dreaming.

CHAPTER 11
TREATING PTSD LUCIDLY

*'Trauma is hell on Earth. Trauma
resolved is a gift from the gods.'*

Peter A. Levine,
developer of Somatic Experiencing®

Sometimes a person enters our life who changes everything. At the time we may not see it, but years later we realize that if we hadn't met that particular person, our life wouldn't be what it is now.

One of those people for me was Keith McKenzie, a veteran of the British army's elite Parachute Regiment as well as a retired firefighter with 20 years' service. It was through Keith that I started working with military veterans and people experiencing post-traumatic stress disorder (PTSD).

Clinically speaking, PTSD is a disabling psychiatric disorder that can occur after exposure to a traumatic event. Trauma is the effect of any stressful experience that overwhelms a person's ability to cope and to integrate their response to that stressful experience. The main symptoms of PTSD can be anxiety, panic attacks, flashbacks, depression and nightmares. In fact, nightmares are one of the hallmarks of PTSD, with between 50 and 70 per cent of people with clinical PTSD experiencing them.

Psychologically speaking, post-traumatic stress is a totally normal response to a traumatic experience. As we go through a traumatic incident, almost all of us will experience a high level of distress and fear. This has an 'aftershock' effect on our nervous system, which might result in nightmares, anxiety, depression or feeling scared to revisit the place where the incident occurred or to do the activity that led to the trauma. This is a hardwired part of our physiology and totally natural.

Charlie says

'I personally feel that the use of the word "disorder" in the PTSD acronym is unhelpful and that we should replace it with the word "display". Post-traumatic stress isn't a disorder or a pathology, it's a totally natural display of the body and mind in response to what has happened to us.'

I first met Keith at a place where wild horses roam and all killing is prohibited, a sanctuary for both nature and spirituality called Holy Isle, a tiny island off the coast of Arran, Scotland, stewarded by my Buddhist teacher Lama Yeshe Rinpoche. Keith was attending the annual Holy Isle lucid dreaming retreat and he had quite a breakthrough, as he was able to, in his words, 'integrate more of my PTSD in that four-day retreat than in four years of therapy'.

A few years later, when Keith had become a fully trained mindfulness meditation teacher and armed forces Buddhist chaplain, he asked me if I would come to one of the mindfulness retreats that he had organized for military veterans and teach them the lucid dreaming techniques that had worked for him. I had no idea whether they would work for other veterans, but it turned out that they did.

Inspired by that first retreat, Keith helped me to begin working with more veterans' groups and then with serving military personnel too. In 2018 this led me to secure a Winston Churchill Memorial Trust Fellowship to research best practice in mindfulness-based approaches to PTSD. The research took me to the USA and Canada to study and train with some of the leading organizations in the field and I ended up presenting my findings at a mindfulness symposium at the British Ministry of Defence in London.

Since then I've been running lucid dreaming and mindful sleep workshops for military veterans, serving military, blue-light service personnel and other groups who have high levels of trauma.

Charlie says

'My fourth book, Wake Up to Sleep, is aimed at people struggling with sleep and contains the breathwork, NSDR (non-sleep, deep rest), Yoga Nidra and sleep awareness practices that I offer at these workshops. Please do check it out if you are suffering from stress or trauma-affected sleep.'

The IONS Study

In 2020 I was approached by a molecular biologist called Dr Garret Yount at the Institute of Noetic Sciences (IONS) in California, who had heard of my work with military veterans and wanted to find out if lucid dreaming could be used not just to treat nightmares, but full-blown post-traumatic stress disorder. Was it possible to actually reduce people's waking-state PTSD symptoms through lucid dreaming? Could we prove that lucid dreaming could not only reduce nightmares but also symptoms such as flashbacks, anxiety and panic attacks?

It had never been done before, so although I was open-minded, I was also unsure. I had never worked with a group in which *everybody* had chronic PTSD and I had never had my methods scientifically scrutinized before.

How Did the Study Actually Work?

The pilot study consisted of 55 participants, all of whom had chronic PTSD and met the clinical criterion for PTSD diagnosis using the self-report PTSD Checklist for DSM-5 symptom criteria. Some participants were survivors of childhood sexual abuse, whereas others were military veterans, with two-thirds of participants being female and most hailing from either the USA or the UK.

With lockdown scuppering our in-person plans, the study ended up being a six-day online lucid dreaming workshop taught by me, consisting of 22 hours of live instruction via Zoom, in which the participants were taught lucid dream induction techniques and how to use lucid dreaming to transform their nightmares and to integrate their trauma.

PTSD and trauma nightmares are disempowering experiences but to become fully aware within a nightmare and know that it's just a dream is a deeply empowering experience that leads to intense feelings of relief and allows the underlying psychological trauma to be released and integrated at a neurological level.

Due to the entire group having chronic PTSD, James Scurry, a UK-based UKCP-accredited psychotherapist, was present at all times during the workshop and was available for one-to-one check-ins at any time throughout the study.

Our main aim was for the participants to become lucid in their dreams and to intentionally use their lucid dreams to transform their nightmares and to integrate their trauma.

At the start of the week, all the participants completed the PTSD Checklist (PCL-5), which is a 20-item questionnaire corresponding to the DSM-5 symptom criteria for PTSD, and the Nightmare Experience Scale, a medical model for measuring nightmare intensity and frequency.

At the end of the week, they completed the same questionnaires, and then four weeks later, they took them again. This, along with daily data collection about their dreams, formed the core of the collected data and results.

The study proved lucid dreaming was one of the most effective and non-invasive, non-addictive, non-medical treatments for post-traumatic stress disorder currently available, while confirming its reputation as one of the most powerful ways of transforming nightmares and trauma while we sleep.

Before we explore the almost unbelievable results, let's look at exactly how the participants integrated their trauma through their lucid dreams.

Dream Planning to Heal Trauma

Almost all of the lucid dreaming techniques found in this book were taught to the participants, but the core and most vital technique was Dream Planning (see page 73).

Each participant had a personally tailored dream plan that they would then enact within their first or next lucid dream.

Some of them made plans to call out affirmations of healing intent or to meet internal archetypes such as the wounded inner child or shadow, while some simply planned to intentionally stay in their recurring nightmare, witnessing it rather than running from it, while reminding themselves: 'My body is safe in bed, I am dreaming, I am safe, I am ready to bear witness.'

One participant, who was working with chronic pain as part of her PTSD symptoms, became lucid and called out, 'Dreamer, heal my body!' and then immediately experienced her body vibrating with healing energy of such force that it was roaring through her ears.

One female participant became lucid and called out to meet her inner lioness (her archetype of protection and power) and spent the lucid dream being guided around the dream under the lioness's protection.

She said, 'For the first time ever I felt safe in my dreams. I woke feeling refreshed, relieved, hopeful and so inspired. I've gone from dreading sleep to looking forward to my dreams now. What an incredible gift!'

Another, who was working with debilitating anxiety, requested to meet and befriend her anxiety within the lucid dream, and when she did, a giant golden throat lozenge appeared and she entered into a state of amazement and felt deep gratitude towards this symbol of healing.

Charlie says

'If this were my dream,[1] I would see the throat lozenge made of gold as a symbol of precious healing and the spontaneous experience of awe and gratitude as not only the transformation of anxiety, but also the understanding that it was actually just trying to keep me safe.'

With so many of the participants having complex PTSD, including many of those who had suffered childhood sexual trauma, we found that making a dream plan to meet and heal the inner child was one of the most popular and most powerful techniques.

I advised participants against calling out to meet their childhood trauma directly in the lucid dream and suggested that they invoke their inner child instead, as it was this part of themselves that had been wounded by the trauma and so provided a crucial buffer zone between the past trauma and the present traumatized experience.

Those who did this were often met with a symbolic representation of their wounded inner child (a crying little girl in one instance), whom they could then embrace with love and kindness.

Retraumatization?

The Dalai Lama famously said, 'If you can't help, then at least don't harm,' and it's a maxim that lies at the core of my work, especially my work with traumatized populations.

Some people may be concerned that intentionally facing and embracing their trauma in a lucid dream could risk retraumatization. Thankfully, this is an unwarranted concern. As we learned earlier, dreaming about painful events actually helps reduce the negative effects of difficult memories, and REM dreaming has been purpose-built through evolution to safely explore and integrate trauma. Through lucid dreaming, we are simply facilitating that process consciously and, crucially, allowing it to happen in a brain that will actually integrate the trauma just as it would if we were awake. Also, once we're lucid, our brain simply won't allow us to do retraumatizing things: just as it will automatically pull back our hand from a fire, it will either wake us up or simply block our request if we try to do something harmful in a lucid dream.

For the pioneer of shadow integration, psychiatrist Carl Jung, this was an intelligent self-regulation mechanism in the psychic apparatus that strove to maintain balance within the mind. I have seen this mechanism in action dozens of times, both in my own lucid dreams and those of others. Whether the mind simply ignores the request to meet the trauma or puts up a flashing neon sign saying: 'Access denied' (that actually happened to a friend of mine), there's no way that it will let us go too far.

The Mechanisms of Trauma Integration through Lucid Dreaming

Although scientists aren't fully aligned on exactly how trauma integration through lucid dreaming actually works at a neurological level, here are the top four hypotheses.

Brain Chemistry

There is a stress chemical called noradrenaline, also known as norepinephrine, that is almost always present in the brain in low amounts, but completely absent during REM sleep. This is so that when we dream about traumatic experiences, we can process the upsetting memories in a 'safe space' free from stress hormones. Sleep scientist Dr Els van der Helm explains that 'During REM sleep, painful memories are being reactivated and integrated, but this all happens in a state where stress neurochemicals are beneficially suppressed.'[2] However, in some people with chronic PTSD, the level of noradrenaline in their brain is markedly higher at all times, including when they dream, meaning that when they do so, they are dreaming in a space that has not been 'made safe'. These high levels of noradrenaline during REM prevent the healing quality of the nightmares that occur within it. And so, for people with high levels of PTSD, nightmares may be more like retraumatizing flashbacks than therapeutic interventions.

But if they can become lucid in their nightmares, there is a massive drop in those stress hormone levels as they realize that they are actually dreaming and not in any real danger. Essentially, the act of becoming lucid significantly lowers stress hormone levels in the brain, thus allowing the healing capacity of the REM dream state to be engaged once more.

Although not yet widely accepted, I believe that this is the underlying biological mechanism of how lucid dreaming helps cure PTSD nightmares, and preliminary studies involving stress hormone saliva samples taken before and after a healing lucid dream have shown this to be the case.

The Brain Thinks We're Awake

And, as we learned earlier, as our neurological system doesn't differentiate between waking and lucid dream experiences, if we face a fear or integrate a trauma in a lucid dream, our brain thinks that we have actually done so in real life and so will rewire its neural connections to reflect this.

This is the real crux of lucid dreaming as far as trauma integration goes: rewiring the brain while we sleep.

Prefrontal Cortex Activation

The renowned trauma specialist Dr Bessel van der Kolk famously stated that for trauma to be fully integrated, the part of the brain that had been knocked offline by the traumatic experience (the prefrontal cortex) had to be brought back online, while the part of the brain that had been dysregulated (the amygdala) had to be regulated.

Facing a trauma in the lucid dream state ticks both these boxes, as it contains the reactivation of the prefrontal cortex (as we become lucid) and the regulation of the amygdala (as we pro-actively transmute and integrate our trauma).

Stuck Record Theory

Due to the elevated stress hormone levels mentioned above, in some cases the brain is unable to use REM sleep to integrate the traumatic memories as usual and so will attempt the integration process over and over again, getting stuck on a loop like a broken record. This is what leads to recurring nightmares.

The simple act of becoming lucid and intentionally staying in the nightmare (rather than trying to wake up) can often be enough in and of itself to 'lift the needle' on the stuck record and integrate the underlying trauma. How? By allowing the nightmarish manifestation of trauma to express itself and be consciously witnessed, we are allowing that energy to be seen, released and integrated.

Almost Unbelievable Results

Whatever the underlying mechanism actually is, though, the results speak for themselves: the vast majority of participants in the study experienced 'a remarkable decrease in PTSD symptoms within I week' through using lucid dreaming alone.

In fact, 85 per cent of the participants showed such a significant decrease that they were no longer classified as having PTSD (using the self-report PTSD Checklist for DSM-5).

The plummeting line on the graph below shows just how drastic the decrease in PTSD symptoms was. It was almost unbelievable.

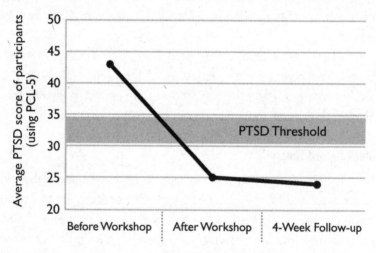

Graph showing reduction of PTSD symptoms after participants attended a lucid dreaming healing workshop.

Lead scientist of the study, molecular biologist Dr Garret Yount, said, 'These results are truly remarkable and highly significant. Immediately following the study, the average PTSD score dropped well below the PTSD symptom threshold and stayed this way four weeks later.'

In 15 years of teaching lucid dreaming, I have never seen such outstanding results for any lucid dreaming study, let alone one as ambitious as this was. Although it was just a 55-person pilot study, the results were so impressive that the team and I have since completed a 100-person randomized control study, which is the golden standard for research.

The data from this larger study (which followed almost exactly the same protocol) will be published in late 2024, but I am happy to say that we replicated the results again under control conditions and the vast majority of the test group displayed such a significant drop in PTSD symptoms that they were also no longer classed as having PTSD.

Without doubt, both the pilot study and the follow-up 100-person study show lucid dreaming to be one of the most powerful treatments for PTSD currently available.

And yet, lucid dreaming for trauma treatment is still relatively unknown within the therapeutic community, which is why in 2019 I started offering Lucid Dream Facilitator Training courses to psychotherapists, medical doctors, meditation teachers, healers and trauma specialists. Visit www.charliemorley.com for details of the next training courses and join me to help bring the transformative benefits of lucid dreaming to those who need them most.

CHAPTER 12
BLURRING THE BOUNDARIES

*'Deep into that darkness peering, long I stood
there, wondering, fearing, doubting, dreaming
dreams no mortal ever dared to dream before.'*

Edgar Allan Poe

The lucid dream is a unique state of consciousness in which we gain access to a depth of mind unfathomable to people who haven't yet experienced it. And once lucid, we can use our increased energetic capacity as a springboard to dive through the boundaries of the dream into something quite different.

Moving through these boundaries is part of the germination of the practice. We descend into the depths of our own mind, and if we keep on swimming deeper and deeper down, we may find that the boundary between our personal consciousness and universal consciousness begins to blur.

Freud famously popularized the iceberg theory of consciousness, in which a small percentage of our mind is above the surface, conscious and tangible, and the majority below the surface, unconscious and rarely accessible. Through lucid dreaming, we not only gain access to the vast expanse of the iceberg below the surface, but also to the infinite sea of awareness in which the iceberg floats.

So, if we travel to the outer limits of a lucid dream we may find a partially permeable membrane through which we can access states beyond our personal mindstream. Through a form of conscious osmosis we can leave the limitations of our own mind behind and flow into the limitless awareness of the void, which gives rise to some extraordinary phenomena.

Prophetic Dreams

> *'A dreamer is one who can only find his way by*
> *moonlight, and his punishment is that he sees*
> *the dawn before the rest of the world.'*
> **Oscar Wilde**

Within Tibetan Buddhism, prophetic dreams are classed as a type of clarity dream and have been systematically used by realized masters to help find reincarnations and to inform themselves of future events. Nevertheless, for the most part it's believed that 'although certain prophecies of future happenings may be true, mostly they will not be'[1] and that to believe that all of your dreams are prophetic is often a sign of an overactive ego. So it is advised within the Buddhist teachings to check your motivation carefully before you claim to have had a prophetic dream.

In the West, prophetic dreams have been close to our heart since our culture began. In fact the propagation of Christianity into the West can be attributed in part to a prophetic dream. The Roman emperor Constantine dreamed of the cross on the night before a big battle and then attributed his victory to the dream.[2] Apparently this led him to make Christianity the new religion of the Roman Empire.

More recently, both Freud and Jung acknowledged dream telepathy.[3] In *Man and his Symbols*, Jung comments that the unconscious has a facility to predict future events, not due to any mystical aptitude but rather to the vast amount of information it stores:

> *Dreams sometimes announce certain situations long before they actually happen. This is not necessarily a form of precognition... What we fail to see consciously is frequently perceived by our unconscious, which can pass the information on through dreams.*[4]

It is as if the data that the unconscious stores (but the conscious mind ignores) can be used to create predictive algorithms of possible future outcomes. Sometimes these predictions come true. This is not necessarily precognition, more like preparation.

Over a third of British people claim to have had at least one dream that prophesied a future event,[5] and although there is a lot of research that disproves most seemingly prophetic dreams as contrived coincidences noticed after the actual event, there is just too much data in favour of prophetic dreams to ignore them completely.

In the 2022 book *The Premonitions Bureau* we learn that in the late 1960s John Barker, a 42-year-old British psychiatrist, started a project called the Premonitions Bureau, where people would send their prophetic dreams. The bureau staff read through hundreds of dreams. Most of them weren't prophetic, but some absolutely were. Barker wanted to 'present the Bureau's findings to the Medical Research Council, with a view to setting up an official national early warning system',[6] but alas, it was not to be.

In 1997 a paper published in the *Journal of the American Society for Psychical Research* proved that 37 of a supposed 51 precognitive dreams gathered for the study could be objectively substantiated.[7] Throughout my own research into this topic I've been shocked by just how much scientific data there is supporting the possibility of prophetic dreams.

Among the most memorable were two cases presented at the Scientific and Medical Network conference at Winchester University in 2011. One was that of an American woman who kept dreaming that she had breast cancer, even though scans found nothing. She eventually paid for invasive surgery and a tiny cyst was found, too small to show up on the scan, that had all the hallmarks of turning malignant in the future.[8] Then there was the case of a group of stock market investors led by a dream psychologist called Arthur Bernard, who ended up making a sales profit of US$1.6 million in 1998 (over US$3 million in today's money) after one of them had a prophetic dream about buying shares in an obscure biotech firm.[9] In the words of one of the presenters at the conference, Dr Larry Dossey, 'We are way beyond anecdotes here, the evidence is just too strong to ignore.'[10]

Charlie says

'I know what you're probably thinking: If people can have dreams of the future, why don't they dream of the winning lottery numbers? Well, actually they do! In one well-documented example, a woman in America won the lottery twice after dreaming of the winning numbers!'[11]

Prophetic dreams can be split into two main categories:

1. Precognitive dreams (pre = before, cognitive = knowing)

2. Premonition dreams (pre = before, monition = warning).

But how do they actually work?

Dr Larry Dossey, a well-known pioneer of science-based research into spirituality, considers that we may well be genetically endowed for premonition dreams, as they would seem to aid our survival.[12] He believes that prophetic dreams may be a type of innate but often dormant preventative medicine that resides within all of us, and he even cites examples in which his stint as a Vietnam War surgeon led to a series of premonition dreams, some of which even saved his life.

The Nobel Prize-winning physicist Brian Josephson says, 'It's not clear in physics why we *can't* see the future,'[13] and although frustratingly inconclusive, the closest to a scientific explanation we have for prophetic dreams is that they may be caused by our consciousness engaging in non-local communication through the vast quantum interconnectivity of reality, in which time, and thus past and future events, are relative. Nobody knows for sure, but then nobody knows for sure what dark energy is either, and that makes up 70 per cent of the known universe.[14] Perhaps for now we will have to accept that although we don't have a cast-iron explanation for how this phenomenon works, we do have some pretty convincing examples that it does work.

Since writing the first edition of this book, I have gained my own pretty convincing example too. In 2018 I fought as the co-main event at a kickboxing show in London and, in the weeks leading up to the fight, I had a very specific dream in which I badly hurt my opponent. When I saw the damage I had caused, I dropped to my knees and bowed in front of him in apology. This dream really got stuck in my head and I couldn't shake the sense of foreboding that it gave me. It really affected my confidence, but I never thought that it could be prophetic.

At the fight itself it was actually me who got badly injured (a broken nose from an accidental head-butt) rather than my opponent, but you can clearly see in the video that my opponent drops to his knees in front of me when he realizes what he has done, just as I did in the dream. This is such an unexpected thing to do that his coach can be heard yelling at him to get up, but it did happen nonetheless, almost exactly as I had seen in my dream.

How Can We Encourage Prophetic Dreams?

It has been said that: 'Premonitions are our birthright. Our capacity for them is part of our original equipment, something that comes factory installed.'[15] So, if precognitive dreams are natural, why don't most of us have them regularly?

The reason may be because most of us aren't in tune with our own nature or our own dreams, so we aren't tuned into the wavelength on which they are broadcast. Some people believe that our natural capacity for precognitive dreaming has deteriorated due to our use of modern communications technology, which has led to our telepathic muscles atrophying from lack of use, but I believe the truth is more straightforward: our sixth sense has withered not only from lack of use but also from lack of attention. Most people are simply not interested in it.

Once we inhabit the awareness of our subtle energies and sixth-sense capacity through mind-training practices, however, or even simply open ourselves up to the possibility that they exist, we become less disconnected from them and less limited. So, we can help remedy our precognitive dreaming limitations by practising energy work such as kundalini yoga, *tai chi* or *chi gong*, as well as keeping a dream diary in order to pay homage to our dreaming mind. These practices will boost the power of our extra-sensory awareness and deepen our connection to our subtle energies and our dreaming mind.

The unconscious is far more likely to offer a precognitive dream to someone who is already in tune with their dream life than to someone with no dream recall or interest in their dreams. However, the most direct way to open up our potential for precognitive dreaming is to become lucid. Due to the refined level of consciousness we enter into through the lucid dream state, we become more attuned to the innate capacity of our sixth sense, which is often pushed aside in the waking state by the more dominant five senses. As we learned earlier, the lucid dream state is a 'thin' place, meaning that its boundaries are semi-permeable. Remember, the dream yoga teachings say that while lucid, we have seven times the power of mind that we have in the waking state.[16] This means that we can ask for information, which can be invited back through the semi-permeable membrane of the dream state and deciphered with seven times our waking clarity. By intentionally calling out for future information within a lucid dream, I have seen detailed images of people I have yet to meet, been warned of coming family illnesses (which tragically did come to pass) and even received four winning numbers on the lottery.*

If future information can be invited into the lucid dreaming mind, perhaps it can be sent out from it, too? In 2011 I conducted an informal experiment into dream telepathy with the members of the monthly Lucid Dream Drop-in. I was to get lucid sometime within the next 30 nights, visualize the attendees and tell them where on my body I had a birthmark.

Funnily enough, I ended up forgetting about the experiment and it was only on the night before the next month's forum that I remembered it. That night I became lucid, visualized as many of the attendees as I could recollect and then called out, 'Right hip! The birthmark is on my right hip!' I even visualized the birthmark and projected it up into the sky in the lucid dream as I repeated, 'The birthmark is on my right hip!'

The next day I asked the dream forum members if anyone had received a dream or any other indication as to where my birthmark was. After a good minute of silence and polite smiles, I continued, 'OK. Well, not to worry, but the birthmark is actually on…' and then suddenly one of the members, who had been looking through his dream diary, called out, 'Right hip! It's on your right hip, isn't

---

* I gave the money I won to charity. In fact, that was part of deal, because when I went into the lucid dream I called out, 'Give me the winning lottery numbers! If I win, I'll give the money to charity!'

it? I think it might be on your right ankle, but the dream says it's definitely on your right hip.'*

But all this is for nothing unless we have some way of telling if this dream information is the real deal, right? How do we know?

It is said that although the vast majority of dreams aren't premonition dreams, if you do have one it will leave such a lasting mental and possibly even somatic remnant afterwards that you'll be in no doubt about it.[17] Remember, precognitive dreams may be a kind of evolutionary trait, so your gut instinct will be really trying to make sure that you get the warning message. Also, the dream will seem very different from the dreams you've had before and it may recur until you've taken on board its message.[18]

Premonition dreams are undoubtedly weird boundary experiences, but not nearly as weird as our next subject...

Out-of-Body Experiences (OBEs)

'I don't think that we're in Kansas anymore, Toto...'
Dorothy, The Wizard of Oz

An out-of-body experience (sometimes referred to as astral projection) typically involves the subjective separation or dislocation of personal consciousness from the physical body. This often allows the consciousness or sense of self to explore not only physical waking reality but seemingly alternate dimensions as well.

Although there are dozens of variations, the classic OBE involves our sense of self shifting out of our physical body and looking back to see it lying below. This type of dislocation of consciousness has been well documented and medically verified as a neurological

---

* Weirdly, I do actually have a mole on my right ankle.

response to shock, intense stress, trauma or anaesthetic, and yet full OBEs have yet to be accepted by mainstream science.

Scientific studies in 2010 have shown that the idea that our sense of self is fixed in our body is a misconception anyway. If the body's sense of spatial awareness is sufficiently confused by receiving contradictory input, then the sense of self will locate itself in a close but separate location to the body.

The study that best proved this point was run by researchers at the Karolinska Institute in Stockholm.[19] They conducted an experiment aimed at creating the illusion, and physical sensation, of having a third arm. In five separate laboratory experiments, 154 volunteers were seated with their hands on a table and a rubber arm placed next to their right arm. A sheet covered their shoulders and elbows, creating the illusion that they had three arms. The scientists then gently brushed the real and fake hands at the end of those arms. Sometimes the brushing occurred simultaneously, sometimes separately. When it occurred at the same time, the subjects would report feeling the sensation in the rubber hand as well and even feeling as if they had two right hands. Their sense of personal self had partially left or at least expanded from the constraints of their physical body to include an inanimate object, the fake rubber arm. There are some great videos of this online. Just search for the 'rubber hand illusion'.

You might be thinking, *If we can relocate the conscious awareness of a limb to outside ourselves, could we do so with our entire body?* It seems that we can, as researchers in France have used the rubber arm experiment to inspire a kind of rubber body experiment that has demonstrated that 'there is a systematic relationship between the body-part illusion and full-body illusion',[20] which allows the sense of self to relocate into another *full-body* form.

Although these experiments are more indicative of bodily illusions than OBEs, they are still an interesting way to show that although our consciousness is *habitually* limited to our physical body, it is not *exclusively* limited.

But what I'd like to focus on now is the kind of intentional OBE or 'astral projection' that most often occurs in or around the boundaries of falling asleep and dreaming: a sleep-initiated OBE.* In these experiences beginners sometimes feel intense rushing vibrations as they pass through the hypnagogic or hypnopompic sleep states and experience their consciousness being separated, often forcibly, from their physical body. Once their consciousness has been separated, they might find themselves in an energy duplicate of their body or sometimes as a point of awareness seemingly floating around anywhere from their local environment to an apparently alternate reality. But are they really dislocated from their physical body or are they just imagining it all?

There is quite an argument for the possibility that the only difference between a night-time 'OBEer' and a lucid dreamer is that the lucid dreamer knows that they're inside their own mind, whereas the OBEer believes that they are experiencing a reality outside themselves. Some researchers believe that most sleep-initiated OBEers are simply lucid dreamers who haven't become fully lucid yet.

Dream researcher Paul Devereux believes that it is very simple: lucid dreamers know that they are experiencing a dream within their mind, while those who label the experience an OBE take the dream to be waking reality.

Another argument that the sceptics throw in is that in sleep-initiated OBEs in which the subject seems to be experiencing actual waking reality (sometimes called a 'Locale I' OBE), they are really just experiencing a false awakening. In a false awakening we

---

* 'Sleep-initiated OBE' is a bit of a misnomer because in some cases the subjects are more in a state of heightened awareness than a sleep state, but it seems the best label to use here nonetheless.

often find ourselves in a mentally constructed carbon copy of our sleeping area that seems to all intents and purposes to be waking reality. But if we become lucid within a false awakening, we recognize that although it may look exactly like waking reality we are in fact still inside our own head.

I used to be an OBE sceptic myself, actually – until I had my first proper OBE, that is. I was sure that most OBEs were just a type of unrecognized lucid dream, and in fact I still believe that many people are mixing up the two, but once I had experienced proper OBEs (both through transition into sleep and while wide awake), I realized that the only reason some people might be confused about the difference between a lucid dream and an OBE was that they hadn't had sufficient experience of either one.

So let's take a closer look at OBEs and see how they form one of the best-documented aspects of consciousness exploration yet to be accepted by mainstream science.

Proof of OBEs

B. Alan Wallace once said, 'If there is just one evidential OBE then that's all you need to know. If you find one white crow, then there are white crows. You don't need to find 100, one is enough.'[21] But have we really found that one white crow yet?

Much of the proof of OBEs being the real deal (and not just some sort of dream phenomenon) comes not from the mystics who are claiming to have them, but from the scientists who are trying to disprove them.

Scientifically speaking, lucid dreams and OBEs are psychologically and physiologically distinct. In the early eighties the Australian professor Harvey Irwin conducted a thorough comparative study[22] of lucid dreams and sleep-initiated OBEs that concluded that most OBEs were unlike lucid dreams because during an OBE the brainwave patterns would often show alpha activity but hardly ever any REM, meaning that whatever the subjects were actually doing, they were definitely not dreaming.

To add to this neuroscientific evidence, we can offer the sceptics some more from scientifically oriented psychology. Keith Harary, executive director of the Institute for Advanced Psychology in Portland, Oregon, has done some excellent all-round OBE studies. Although he still believes that nobody actually knows quite what an OBE is, he proved under scientific conditions that his pet cat displayed significantly more settled behaviour when he had guided his sense of self to its location during several randomly timed OBEs than when his sense of self (or whatever he believed was being projected out of his body) was not with the cat.

But what about the physicists? Surely they can't believe in all this stuff? On the contrary, some of the most convincing experiments into OBEs were conducted by a nuclear physicist called Dr Thomas Campbell. In his book *My Big TOE*, Campbell describes the process through which he validated his OBEs:

> *Somebody would write down a random number and we would read it while our bodies lay asleep. Then they would erase it and write another one, and so on and on. We went places – to people's homes – and saw what they were doing, then called them or talked to them the next day to check it out for validation.*[23]

Campbell collected some of the most convincing data for the OBE as a real phenomenon distinct from sleep, and his position as a respected nuclear physicist gave his data even more kudos.

And then of course there is the work of Robert Monroe. If you still have any doubts about the validity of OBEs after reading this chapter, then read his seminal work, *Journeys Out of the Body*. In this, he describes dozens of personal accounts of OBEs meticulously analysed for inconsistencies and far too detailed to be the work of a fraud.

Monroe went on to set up the non-profit Monroe Institute, which gathered so much hard proof of the validity of OBEs that the former director of the Intelligence and Security Command of the US Army sent his personnel there for training. I know that seems hard to believe, but it's true. In fact, US Army documents declassified in 1995 reveal that the US government invested millions of dollars over 20 years in several top-secret projects such as the Stargate project (well worth a google) which aimed to use OBEs and remote viewing as a way of spying on the Russian military during the Cold War. One of these 'psychic spies', a man named Joe McMoneagle, was even awarded the Legion of Merit by the US military for his discovery of a Russian submarine in 1979 through remote viewing.

Although there is no conclusive agreement on how they happen, OBEs arising from stress, trauma or anaesthesia have been verified, so why is it so hard for us to believe that they could be induced at will or via the gateway of sleep? For years scientists believed that lucid dreaming was 'a paradoxical impossibility' and that it was in fact just a misdiagnosed form of micro-awakening. Perhaps the argument that a sleep-initiated OBE is simply a misinterpreted dream phenomenon is just as weak?

We cannot dismiss the hundreds of verified accounts from people who have been able to project their consciousness out of their physical body just because we haven't agreed on the scientific explanation for how they've done it. That's exactly what we did with lucid dreamers, meditators and self-hypnotists before Western science eventually caught up with them.

The scientific evidence for OBEs is just too overwhelming to ignore, but even without it there are many discernible differences between OBEs and lucid dreams that we can use to differentiate the two.

> ## Charlie says
>
> 'Lucid dreams require that the subject is in REM dreaming sleep, but OBEs can be engaged from the waking state. In fact, you don't even need to be lying down to have an OBE, let alone be asleep. My friend the OBE researcher Graham Nicholls told me of an OBE he had once that began while he was walking into his kitchen. He felt the energy shift begin as he entered his kitchen, and as it increased, he lay down on the floor to allow the full experience to manifest.'

How to Spot an OBE

I've had hundreds of lucid dreams over the past 20 years, so I know the lucid dream state well enough to know when I'm in it and when I'm not. When I have an OBE, I'm definitely not in the lucid dream state as I know it. They feel as different as water and ice – the same essence perhaps, but totally different forms.

The entry into an OBE is often very different from that of a lucid dream. If you enter the OBE state through the transition into sleep (much like the FAC technique), rather than the gradual layering of the hypnagogic imagery, you may experience intense vibrations, loud audio hallucinations and a rushing sensation as your consciousness is forcibly shifted out of your body. When you first experience this, you'll be in no doubt that you're not entering a lucid dream.

How can you tell that you're not merely in another lucid dream? Because reality checks and other lucid dream indicators won't function in the same way.*

---

* It may seem that entry into an OBE from the lucid dream state is the best argument *against* OBEs being distinct from lucid dreams, but in fact this technique can be a great way to cross-reference the many differences between the two phenomena.

In a lucid dream we can change aspects of the dreamscape because we're inside our personal mindstream, but in an OBE it's much more difficult to change things, because we aren't in our personal mindstream, we're in a shared one. In lucid dreams, gravity is relative to expectation, but in an OBE, the 'expectation effect' is out of the window because it isn't our mental expectations that are creating the environment.

Also, in most lucid dreams, we are embodied: we have a body with which we explore the dream. This body is a mental projection, of course, just like everything else in the lucid dream. In an OBE, however, we may not have a body at all, and if we do, it may be translucent. Or we may be just a point of awareness. This allows us to look at our physical body while we are out of it.

And finally, in lucid dreams, time is relative to waking time (laboratory studies have found that a five-minute lucid dream feels subjectively as though it has taken five minutes[24]), but in the OBE state, time is very different. What may feel like a four-hour OBE can turn out to have lasted only 20 minutes. This is a subtle but profound difference between the two.

As you can see, there are many different ways to tell the difference between an OBE and a lucid dream, but the easiest way to get to grips with these differences is to spend as much time as possible in these states. I still believe that there are loads of people who are mistakenly labelling pre-lucid dreams and false awakenings as OBEs, but I now know beyond all doubt that in a true OBE experience you can intentionally leave your personal mindstream and the limitations of your own head.

The Tibetan Buddhist View on OBEs

In Tibetan Buddhism, both lucid dreaming and OBE work are found within the dream yoga practices. Lama Yeshe Rinpoche once described the difference between the two phenomena in very simple terms: 'Lucid dreaming? In your head. But, also, you can go out of your head!'

Those of you who are typically sceptical Buddhists, please relax those pursed lips and furrowed brows at this point, for it should be noted that the practice of separating the subtle energy body from the gross corporeal body has a long tradition in Tibetan Buddhism.* In fact even the wonderfully solid Akong Rinpoche once told me, 'Learning astral projection will be of benefit in the *bardo* state because that separation of the body and mind is exactly what happens in the after-death *bardo*. If you can learn the basics of this then, yes, that will be useful.'[25]

The Tibetan dream yoga teachings refer to the body that we have in lucid dreams as the 'dream body' and the one that we have in our out-of-body astral travels as the 'special dream body'.

In *Sleeping, Dreaming, Dying*, the brilliant dialogue between neuroscience and Buddhism, HH Dalai Lama says: 'The special dream body is created from the mind and from vital energies (*prana*) within the body. It is able to disassociate from the gross physical body and travel elsewhere. This is not just imagination; the subtle self actually departs from the gross physical body.'[26]

Andrew Holecek, author of the seminal book *Dream Yoga*, expands: 'The special dream body can be projected to different places. The special dream body can observe physical beings, but most physical beings cannot see the special dream body.'[27]

Being able to project an aspect of our consciousness from our body was useful in ancient Tibet (it's the size of western Europe) because it offered the ability to receive teachings from inaccessible geographical locations as well as from other realms of existence.

---

* Mindrolling Rinpoche, the renowned Tibetan lama who died in 2008, spent the last few years of his life in an almost constant state of lucid dreaming and astral projection, often practising dream yoga all day, projecting out of his body and interacting with waking reality.

There is no doubt about the difference between lucid dreams and special dream body experiences, and in fact dream yoga practitioners are actively encouraged to check the veracity of their experience not only to differentiate it from a possible lucid dream but also to gain an understanding of emptiness – the pure potentiality of the dreamlike nature of reality.

One of the last teachings that I received from the late great Akong Tulku Rinpoche was an instruction on astral projection: 'Leave body and go into street. Check numbers on houses. Then, next day you go with pen and paper and check numbers.'

Another lama, known as Drupon Rinpoche, instructed me to: 'Look back at your sleeping body. Make sure you see your sleeping body' while in the OBE state.

He encouraged this because by looking back at our body we begin to break the shackles of ego-grasping as we see that we are not limited to our bodily form (and the illusory ego that is so attached to it).

I should add that the separation of the subtle energy body from the gross physical body, which we find in some advanced Tibetan Buddhist meditations, is only ever taught within the safety of a retreat environment and under the guidance of a qualified master, unlike the New Agey 'OBE weekends' that we find offered in the West. Having an OBE can be an incredibly intense experience, and so from a Buddhist point of view it is advised that you only engage the practice once you are well grounded in meditation and compassion training.

OBEs and Lucid Dreams for Spiritual Growth

So, if OBEs allow us to leave our personal mindstream and the limitations of our own head, is lucid dreaming just a stepping stone towards the more advanced practice of astral projection?

I don't think so. When we lucid dream, we are inside our own mind, a place where we can work directly with our own personal psychology, a laboratory for enlightened action in which we can reprogram our negative habitual tendencies for the benefit of both ourselves and all beings, creating new patterns of positive mind states that will profoundly affect the way we think and act. Lucid dreaming makes us kinder, wiser and more awake.

Similarly, OBEs are amazing tools for growth and going out of body is a brilliant skill to foster alongside lucid dreaming. The big selling point of the OBE experience is that it profoundly shifts our view on reality, even more so than lucid dreaming, because it shows us that we are not limited to our own body and that we have the same quantum potentiality as the atoms that make up that body. And of course, having an OBE greatly reduces our fear of death, because it allows us to have a dress rehearsal before the final show.

But without pure motivation and skilful application, all of this potential can end up being no more than a head trip – a head trip outside your own head.

When we have an OBE, I don't believe that we are always travelling to another physical dimension, I believe that we are more often travelling to another mental dimension, which, although it may seem to be separate from us, is in fact still within the realm of the larger universal mind that both encompasses and lies beyond the subjective limitations of our personal mind.

In fact, the name 'OBE' is quite misleading, because it implies that our consciousness is located somewhere in our body and so when we go beyond our personal mind we have gone 'out of our body', whereas our mind and sense of self were never confined to our body in the first place. Perhaps these experiences should be called 'into mind' rather than 'out of body' because there is no reality that is not dependent, at least in part, on the infinite consciousness of mind.

Charlie says

'Whether we are in our mind or out of our body, my advice is this: don't set up a duality within your spiritual practice. Mistaken duality has got us into enough trouble already in the waking state without us slipping into the same trap in our spiritual practice. However dualistic and separate the alternate dimensions that you visit in an OBE may seem, they are not separate, they are all part of you, and part of your mind in exactly the same way as waking reality is.'

CHAPTER 13
BEYOND LUCIDITY

'You take the blue pill, the story ends, you wake up in your bed and believe whatever you want to believe. You take the red pill, you stay in Wonderland and I show you how deep the rabbit-hole goes.'

Morpheus, *The Matrix*

Lucid dreaming takes us beyond mere projection and into aspects of mind that are in the frontier lands of consciousness. Once we set out on the path to lucidity, we begin a journey which may profoundly reconfigure not only our perception of our dreams, but our perception of our waking life too.

In this penultimate chapter, let's ride into the frontier lands and explore the germination of ideas that will challenge our accepted modes of experience and call into question the very nature of waking reality. Let's explore how to wake up from the waking dream and live our life with lucidity as co-creators of the dream of being.

Oneness: The Interconnected Nature of Reality

*'See through the illusion of separateness and
recognize that we are all one... Knowing that
you are one with all, you will find yourself in love
with all, and you will fall in love with living.'*[1]
Gnostic Christian wisdom

Many of the great spiritual traditions tell us that contrary to how we may feel, we are actually in a state of total interdependence, interconnected with all, beyond any notion of separateness. This idea is often referred to as 'Oneness'.

The key motivation for moving towards Oneness is based on the notion that separateness separates us, whereas oneness brings us together, with love, in love. Sounds simple, right? It's a lovely idea and a concept that's easy to understand theoretically, but in practice it can be very hard to see how the 'me, my, I', so distinctly different from 'you', and from the trees and buildings and animals that make up our reality, could ever *not* be separate.

There is, however, a direct way in which to make the theoretical understanding of Oneness experiential: lucid dreaming. Once lucid, we can actually experience the interconnected Oneness that we have heard about, because in a lucid dream we are at one with all things. We are the trees, we are the leaves on the trees, we are the wind that blows through the leaves on the trees. Everything is us and we are everything. And as we enter into the experience of being one with everything, we know that we are dreaming the dream and everything in it into existence. Everything in the dream is part of the projection of our own mind – everything that seems so absolutely real and yet is so absolutely illusory. All aspects of the dream are within our own psyche and so there is no 'us and them', no duality, no separateness, just Oneness.

But it's still just a dream, right? Yes, of course, but once we wake up from a lucid dream in which we've experienced this sense of Oneness, we'll never look at waking reality in quite the same way again. Seeing our inherent Oneness is the beginning of real compassion, because it allows us to reach beyond separation and selfishness.

In a lucid dream, the trees and the people and the buildings look and feel so undeniably separate from us and yet we know that they're not separate because they are all part of our own mind. This knowledge leaves an indelible trace on our waking consciousness that allows us to at least question (and at most directly challenge) the very nature of a waking reality that looks and feels just as separate as the dream did.

Quantum Dreaming

Through the revolution in thought created by the dawn of quantum physics, we now understand that the objective, dualistically existing world is not quite as it seems.

'Quantum physics reveals the basic oneness of the universe'[2] because it shows us that everything is interconnected beyond all notions of separateness, just as it is in a lucid dream. Quantum physics challenges the views of classical physics, which placed us as passive observers in a materialistic universe, because it has proved that we are integrally connected with everything.* But how does this actually work?

If we tap our fingers on a table, for example, it feels solid, and yet it doesn't actually have much substance, because it is made of atoms, and atoms are 99.9999999999 per cent empty space. So, what creates the feeling of solidity? 'Our minds!' shout the

---

* Although quantum theory has been presented in the West as a new idea, in his book *You Are Here*, Christopher Potter shows that it was first explored as far back as the 1700s, when Bishop Berkeley asked if an unobserved tree could be said to exist.

pseudo-science crowd. Well, they're right in part, but it's not quite that simple. Apart from that crucial 0.00000001 per cent that actually does exist, it is the electromagnetic repulsion between the electrons in our fingers and those in the table that stops our fingers passing through it. It is, however, our mind that interprets these electrostatic forces picked up by the pressure sensors in our fingers as the 'feeling of solidity'.*

It has been said that scientific materialism works on the belief that 'there is one indivisible material reality that is universally consistent. Scientists proposing this view believe in a world that can be seen as it actually is: separate from ourselves, out there, a world that can be experienced in exactly the same way no matter where we are in it.'[3] However, as the Nobel Prize-winning physicist Werner Heisenberg said, 'The ontology of materialism rests upon the illusion that the kind of existence, the direct "actuality" of the world around us, can be extrapolated into the atomic range. This extrapolation is, however, impossible.'[4]

This may come as a shocking truth but, as another Nobel Prize-winning physicist Niels Bohr said, 'Those who are not shocked when they first come across quantum theory cannot possibly have understood it.'[5]

Through lucid dreaming we are developing the habit of recognizing the nature of reality and the capacity to directly challenge the illusion of dualistic materialism. This is because once we're lucid, we wake up to the fact that what we previously accepted as reality is actually just a mirage, empty of inherent existence, and, more importantly, we become aware that our consciousness, the observer, is co-creating this dream reality, just as it co-creates our waking reality at a quantum level.

---

* Senior lecturer in chemical psychics Dr Alan Taylor tells me, 'The atoms are held together by electrostatic force and the quantum mechanical phenomenon of bonding. When you push against this electron distribution, it exerts an equal and opposite force back.'

So, lucid dreaming trains us to awaken to the quantum interconnectivity of life. It trains us to recognize the Oneness of waking reality. It trains us for awakening. It has been said that once enlightened, we 'awaken from the dream of being a separate "me" to being the universal reality'[6] and that we wake up to the fact that however dualistic reality seems, there is in fact no 'I' and 'other'. There is no separateness, no division. We are the universal reality of all things, in waking life just as in a lucid dream.

Dreaming our Reality into Existence?

'Those who dream by night wake in the day to find that it was vanity: but the dreamers of the day are dangerous men, for they act out their dreams with open eyes, to make it possible.'
T. E. Lawrence

We now know that an atom only appears in a particular place once we measure it. This means that it is spread out all over the place until a conscious observer decides to look at it. This in turn shows us that the act of observation plays a part in the creation of the universe.

If quantum physics shows us that through the act of observation our consciousness co-creates our reality, then perhaps the quality and intent of our consciousness can affect the creation of that reality?

With so much of experiential reality being governed by our mental outlook, habitual tendencies and personal projection, it doesn't take much to see that in many ways we really are the co-creators of our own reality. 'Two men look out of prison bars; one sees mud, the other sees stars,' as the old saying goes. We are constantly projecting, and this kind of psychological projection is one of the most dominant forces of the human mind – and one that can be transformed into a powerful force of manifestation.

This concept forms the basis of the newly rejuvenated trend for 'manifesting'. We're told by some New Age 'gurus' that if we powerfully visualize getting that new car and set our intent strongly enough, then we will manifest a new car – or nose job, or pay rise, or a host of other samsarically focused goals. These kinds of manifestation practices are actually based on sound spiritual principles that have been unfortunately diluted and repackaged for modern-day consumers.

It takes much more than just making a 'vision board' and really desiring to have lots of money for these things to actually manifest. Just as our level of influence over a lucid dream is only ever that of a co-creator, working alongside the unconscious mind and dependent on our beneficial motivation, so our level of influence over waking life is held within the constraints of the larger universal consciousness. And, vitally, our current experience of waking reality is dictated in large part by the results of our actions, our karma.

Karma: Cause and Effect

Some people don't believe in the hands of fate or a creator God calling the shots on a prearranged future. Instead they believe that they are the masters of their own destiny; they believe in something called karma. Karma is one of the most misunderstood tenets of Eastern spirituality, but one of the most important to understand in view of dreaming our reality into existence.

The word *karma* means 'action', and so with every action of our body, speech and mind, we are creating our future reality. Within us lies the potential to be whatever we choose.

Within Buddhism, 'Karma does not mean punishment. It is the law of cause and effect. If you want to grow a cabbage, then you plant a cabbage seed (cause) and a cabbage grows (effect).'[7] If you plant an acorn hoping for a cabbage, you will end up disappointed, because you will get an oak tree instead. You haven't been *punished* – you are simply experiencing the result of planting a certain seed.

Karma means that we are the masters of our own destiny, because we create our future in the present moment through the seeds we choose to plant. If we want to be happy in the future, we need to plant the seeds of happiness through being kind and helping others. These seeds will then sprout in the form of happiness and beneficial circumstances.

Our karma is of course linked to everybody else's karma, too. The Buddhist nun Pema Chödrön says that because everything is karmically interconnected, 'If you hurt another person, you hurt yourself, and if you hurt yourself, you are hurting another person... We are not in this alone. We are all in this together.'[8]

Our actions count. This is how karma forms the basis not only of our future happiness, but also that of those around us. Karma is the opposite of fate: it means that the future is in our hands because what we do now creates our future.[9] By understanding karma we really can dream our reality into existence, but if we ignore it, we risk our dream becoming a nightmare.

In a lucid dream we are literally dreaming our experiential reality into being because we are influencing and co-creating the dream with our conscious intent. But however skilled we become at this in our dreams, in the waking state we have our karma to deal with too. This means that fervently desiring money or wishing really hard for a new car without carrying out any beneficial action (karma) that might lead to the manifestation of that money or new car is unlikely to have much effect.

The Shared Dream

Albert Einstein once asked Niels Bohr, 'Do you really believe that the moon is not there when nobody looks at it?'

To which Bohr replied, 'Can you prove to me the opposite: that the moon is still there when nobody looks?'

Their interaction makes me wonder: are we really seeing the same reality as everybody else?

The answer is no, not always. The information coming in from our eyes, through the thalamus and into the back of the brain only makes up 10 per cent of the overall information that we use to see.[10] The other 90 per cent comes from other parts of the brain and not from 'out there' at all. This means that what we see through our eyes is only one-tenth of reality and so 'rather than seeing what is physically present, the way we see the world is mostly based upon our prediction of the world'.[11]

People say, 'I'll believe it when I see it!' but it seems that in fact we'll see it when we believe it, because, as neuroscientist Dr Beau Lotto says, 'Seeing is literally believing. We see what we believe.'[12] When the world becomes too familiar, our brain reverts to a kind of 'automatic pilot', which stops seeing what is right in front of our eyes, meaning that for much of the time we're not seeing exactly the same world as everybody else.

It seems that reality is based upon our interaction with it and that our consciousness co-creates our experience of the world. Could lucid dream training help us to learn how to play a part in this creation? The dream yogis seem to think so. The late Traleg Kyabgon Rinpoche said, 'Every time we change our dreams, we increase our capacity to change our conscious experience while we are awake,'[13] and that by training our capacity to direct a lucid dream, we are enhancing our ability to direct the dream of waking reality. This is how lucid dreaming leads to lucid living.

Lucid Living

'Imagine the bliss of becoming lucid at all times, perceiving all things as luminous displays of the deepest dimension of our own awareness. This is the truth that sets us free.'

B. Alan Wallace

For thousands of years Buddhism has proffered that we although we believe that we are awake, our waking lives are actually spent sleepwalking through a dreamlike illusion that we mistake for absolute reality. As we learned earlier, quantum physicists now agree that with only 0.00000000001 per cent of perceived form being something other than space, we partially project mind into form, just as we do in our dreams.

In waking life, however, most of us are still not aware that the majority of reality is a dreamlike illusion and so we feel separate from and threatened by everything that we perceive to be not us. This perceived threat leads to fear and we become afraid of 'the other' and barricade ourselves in against the shock of mistaken dualism.

In a lucid dream, however, we become aware that we are dreaming and 'wake up' to the illusion that what we once thought to be a solid, permanently existing reality is actually just a projection of our own mind. Once we have experienced this awakening, we begin to relax and enjoy the show a bit more in our waking life, because we are aware that it is not quite as solid and inflexible as we have been led to believe.

Every time we lucid dream, we are experiencing a new perception of reality, one in which we are the co-creator, and the more we experience this, the more we may also perceive waking reality in a similar way. Each time we do this, we are creating a habit of recognition. It is this habit of recognizing illusion that forms the crux of lucid living.

Lucid dreamers, empowered by the experiences of their lucid dreams, start to consciously direct and co-create their waking lives, too. They become kinder and more pro-active and discerning in their waking interactions. They embrace the shadow elements of daily life fearlessly* and work through psychological blocks more creatively as they begin to take back the reins of their lives and live more lucidly.

Charlie says

'One of the first people I saw demonstrate lucid living was Robert Waggoner. We had a pint at a pub after one of his dream workshops and he wanted to get a black cab back to his hotel. We were in a residential area of London on a Sunday evening, so I told him that there was no chance of this happening, but he started going on about the interconnectedness of reality and that if we really expected to find a black cab, then we could "intend" one into existence. To be honest, I thought that was just the beer talking, but then suddenly we saw an empty black cab parked outside a house. As we looked at it, a man came out of the house and got into it. He was just starting his shift. Robert looked at me and said, "You see, Charlie, it's all about expectation!"'

How Does It Actually Work?

In a fully lucid dream we experience a boost of awareness that facilitates the realization that we are conscious within our own psyche. This extraordinary awareness reveals that what we thought was separate from us, outside us, apart from us, is in fact inside us and at one with us. Imagine if we could have a similar realization in

---

* Once you've hugged a terrifying shadow monster or turned to face the recurring nightmare that has been haunting you for years, standing up to a bully in the waking state just doesn't seem that scary anymore.

this dream of waking reality. Imagine if we could become lucid while we were awake…

If we want to start having lucid dreams, we need to engage three core principles: strong motivation, effective techniques and, most importantly, a shift in mental perspective that gives us the confidence to believe that lucidity is possible. Similarly, if we engage these three core principles while awake, we can learn to have moments of lucidity in the shared dream of waking life.

Why would we want to become lucid in waking life? Because once we are fully lucid, our human potential is fully realized. In fact, if we were to wake up completely from this dream, we would become a buddha: one who has woken up. Enlightenment is often described as awakening from the dream of being a separate entity to the realization that we are the universal totality of all things.

The more aware and lucid we can be in our daily life, the kinder we can be to ourselves and others. Kindness is the basis of lasting happiness, and we all want to be happy, right? I once asked my teacher Lama Yeshe Rinpoche what the point of being more awake was and he replied with a sentence which I think encompasses the entire spiritual path: 'More awake, more aware. More aware, more kind. More kind: that's the whole point!'[14]

But surely we are awake already? If you're reading this sentence then you must be awake, right? Partially, yes, but just as there are multiple stages of sleep, so there are different stages of wakefulness. It seems strange that we use the word 'awake' to describe everything from pre-sleep drowsiness to post-caffeine alertness. Our entire daily experience is called 'awake' and yet think how it fluctuates. Harvard research has shown that even when we claim to be awake, most of us are unaware, on autopilot or not in the present moment for 47 per cent of our waking life.[15] We may appear to be awake, but we are definitely not fully lucid much of the time.

How Can We Live More Lucidly?

I'm not living lucidly every day of my life, just as I'm not dreaming lucidly every night of my life. But, as with lucid dreaming, which I can do whenever I apply the techniques and put in the effort, I've learned how to have flashes of lucidity in waking life. Here are a few of the techniques that help me live a bit more lucidly.

Meditation

Meditation is one of the original methods for lucid living. It has been found cross-culturally since the Akashic Records began. It may seem a rather paradoxical method: we think that we will keep ourselves awake by constantly doing things, but actually one of the best ways to wake ourselves up is to do nothing – the intentional and very active nothing of mindfulness meditation.

Meditation brings us into direct contact with our inner environment, and through this, we come to know ourselves better and so become better equipped to know when we are on autopilot and when we are truly awake. Meditation is also a form of mind training in which we make our mind stronger, more flexible and healthier. Just as it's impossible to get fit without exercising our body, it's impossible to wake up and live lucidly without exercising our mind.

Mind training is like going to the mind gym; it's about flexing the muscles of our mind to give ourselves the strength to become lucid. Researchers at Harvard, Yale and MIT have found conclusive evidence that regular periods of meditation can actually alter the physical structure of our brain in favour of clarity and lucid awareness.[16] There is no greater tool on the path to lucid living than meditation and I implore you to engage some sort of regular meditation practice if you can. Appendix I (see *page 249*) explains how to practise mindfulness meditation.

Life Signs

As we know, dream signs are aspects of the dream experience that can be used to indicate that we are dreaming. They are triggers that help us become lucid within the dream, but there are also triggers in waking life that can help us become more lucid. I call these 'life signs'.

A life sign is any aspect of our waking experience that reveals the dreamlike nature of reality and helps to wake us from our slumber. Synchronicities, coincidences and flashes of intuition are all potential life signs. Anytime you experience one of these things, be sure to acknowledge it and allow it to wake you up. This is very similar to the Columbo Method that we learned earlier.

The most powerful way to lucid living is to regard waking life as a little bit more dreamlike. Intentionally looking out for life signs will help this shift of perception to take place. This forms the foundation of a Tibetan Buddhist practice called Illusory Body yoga, which is used in conjunction with dream yoga to help the practitioner realize the dreamlike nature of reality.

Be careful not to turn all this into some sort of ego trip, though. Everybody is part of the same dream, so you are no more the central protagonist than anybody else. Having said that, don't be blasé or try to act cool whenever something dreamlike happens. Instead, acknowledge it and be thankful for the opportunity for lucidity.

Charlie says

'English people like myself seem to be the worst at recognizing life signs. If a genie were to pop out of a bottle of beer in an English pub, the most that you'd get from the punters would be a raised eyebrow! But lucid living requires us to notice life signs and allow them to raise our level of awareness, not ignore them out of embarrassment.'

Think about Death More

Buddhist scholar Stephen Batchelor says that one of the paradoxes of the human condition is that 'by meditating on death we become more conscious of life'.[17] Indeed, there is no more visceral way to wake up to life than by thinking about death.

Death is a shared commonality of human experience and yet we never talk about it, at least not in the West. We never discuss it or plan for it or talk about how we would like it to happen. It's as if we think it won't happen at all, and yet we will all die. Definitely.

Charlie says

'Our egoic sense of self dupes us into thinking that if we contemplate death or even mention its name, we will somehow hasten its arrival or jinx ourselves. This is absolute rubbish! Our ego tells us this to maintain its stranglehold over our higher self, and every time we give in to the fear, we feed it, and so its power over us increases.'

Contemplating death wakes us up to both our own potentiality and the limitations of time. Most people have a maximum of 100 years to live their life and offer something of value to the human story. The great master Dilgo Khyentse Rinpoche once said, 'On the day that you were born, you began to die. Do not waste a single moment more!'[18] This sounds extreme, but he knew that mortality awareness helps us to be more motivated, compassionate and lucid.

Contemplating death is a great way to live more lucidly, so I ask you to take a few minutes now to ask yourself this: if you were to die one week from now, would you be able to die at peace with the world? Take time to really contemplate that question, make notes if you like and then see what actions you might be able to carry out to make it possible. Don't wait till you're on your deathbed to make your peace, do it this week while you still have time.

Act Lucidly

I have found that as their practice matures, many lucid dreaming practitioners report that three primary mental attitudes arise within their lucid dreams. These are acceptance, friendliness and kindness.

Acceptance arises from the realization that everything we are seeing, experiencing and interacting with is a projection of our mind and an expression of our own potentiality. Once we have accepted this, we find that friendliness towards everything in the dream arises naturally, because all of it is a part of us. With this friendliness comes a feeling of kindness, as we treat everything in the dream with the kindness with which we would treat ourselves.

If in waking life we truly believed that everything we were seeing, experiencing and interacting with was part of us, just as in a lucid dream, we would find that acceptance, friendliness and kindness arose spontaneously. Unfortunately, this is dependent upon us living lucidly enough to believe it in the first place, which in my experience is easier said than done. But if acceptance, friendliness and kindness arise *from* lucidity in our dreams, perhaps they can *lead to* lucidity in our waking life?

They can and they do. By replicating the mental attitudes of a lucid dream in the waking state, we can create the conditions needed to become lucid in everyday life. To become lucid in life, we just need to start acting lucidly.

....

Let's Act Lucidly!

How do we do that?

Act with acceptance

In this context, 'acceptance' means 'unconditional love towards ourselves and towards all situations in which we find ourselves, however unpleasant they may seem'. It does *not* mean approval or endorsement of negative mind states or situations. It is, however, a prerequisite to actively engaging with negative situations and doing something about them.

If we truly accept not only our present moment, but also that we are interconnected with every single other being in the universe, we will definitely start to live with more love and lucidity.

Act with friendliness
To live lucidly is to approach all situations, good and bad, with unconditional friendliness – that's friendliness towards ourselves, towards others, towards negative emotions, towards change and towards pain. That is the path to lucid living.

Living lucidly is actually impossible without a mental attitude of unconditional friendliness. Why? Because duality is based upon unfriendliness and selfishness. Every time we believe that we are more important than everyone else, we further cement the grasp that duality has over us. But the moment that we see others as equally important or even more important than ourselves (shock horror!), we seem to short-circuit the dreamy dualism of waking life and become more lucid within it.

Act with kindness
Be kind to everything in this life because, just as in a lucid dream, everything is connected to you. Every time we are unkind to someone, we are strengthening the non-lucid belief that we are separate from them. You know that warm feeling after being kind to someone or really helping another person? I believe that warmth is not just the feeling of oxytocin entering the bloodstream, but also the somatic manifestation of lucidity.

Charlie says

'By cultivating acceptance, friendliness and kindness, we stand a far greater chance of living lucidly. Why? Because we're recreating the dominant mind states of fully lucid dreaming while we're awake! It's such a simple idea, but I urge you to try it – it really does help to wake you up.'

We can all live with a little more lucidity, but we have to work at it, just as we do with lucid dreaming. Sometimes we might have flashes of spontaneous lucidity in our waking life, just as we may have spontaneous lucid dreams, but for the most part we need to plan for lucidity. This is fine, of course, but as one Tibetan master commented, 'You like plans, so make your plan, but then put it in your back pocket and live your life in the present moment. Your plan will always be there if you need it.'[19]

Those who practise lucid living aren't procrastinators, they're doers. So, be wise and mindful and don't rush into anything, but at the same time don't get stuck at the planning stage – go out and make things happen. Show the dream that you are ready to co-create it – dance with karma and dream your destiny into existence.

CHAPTER 14
AWAKENING WITHIN THE DREAM

*'To awaken within the dream is our purpose now.
When we are awake within the dream, the ego-
created earth-drama comes to an end and a
more benign and wondrous dream arises.'*

Eckhart Tolle, *A New Earth*

When I was 13, I was sent to an ex-military boarding school. It was a fruitless but compassionate attempt by my parents to get me back onto the rails of discipline. It was there that I not only became interested in philosophy and Buddhism, but also met one of the most curiously intelligent people I had ever come across. He was a wonderfully 'old-school' literature master called Dr Fox, and he once told me a story I have never forgotten – a story about impossibility.

One day when he was a child, sitting at the breakfast table, his mother asked his father for a cigarette. His father reached into his breast pocket, pulled a cigarette from its packet and casually threw it onto the table. It landed not on its side or rolling across the table, but in a perfectly upright position. Dr Fox said that from that day onwards, he knew that nothing was impossible.

That story left an indelible mark on my mind – far more so than the seemingly impossible stories of levitating lamas and clairvoyant gurus that I have heard since. I believe we should be careful before we brand something 'impossible'. It's a lazy label most often used by cynics and sceptics who seem to be the voice of reason – until we discover that there *is* more than one galaxy in our universe and the dream state *can* be experienced consciously.

Lucid dreaming is just one former 'impossibility', which in turn opens the door to further seemingly incredible notions. Whether it's communication with our higher self, lucidly prophesied events or insights into the dream-like nature of waking reality, at some point in our lucidity training we will be challenged to re-evaluate the boundaries of what is possible. It is how we respond to that challenge that counts, because our potential awakening may be dependent upon it.

The central metaphor within Buddhism is that of awakening from a dream. The word *buddha* actually means 'awakened one' and it's said the only difference between us and a fully enlightened buddha is that they have woken up. Woken up from what? From the illusion of separateness, just as we do in a lucid dream.

It's said that sometime after his enlightenment under the bodhi tree, the Buddha was travelling along a road when he encountered a Hindu priest walking towards him. This man was astonished by the Buddha's radiating energy and asked him: 'Are you a god?'

The Buddha replied, 'No.'

'Are you an angel?'

The Buddha again replied, 'No.'

'Are you a spirit then?'

The Buddha replied, 'No.'

The priest tried a fourth time, asking, 'Are you a man?'

Again the Buddha replied, 'No.'

Finally the priest asked, 'Well, what are you then?'

The Buddha replied, 'I am awake.'

The Buddha was neither a god nor an angel nor a spirit; he was a human being who had woken up into a state beyond the limitations of the dualistic self and had made the impossible possible by becoming fully lucid in all states of day and night.

Through lucid dreaming, we can get a taste of this awakening as we experience the extraordinary awareness that we are both within the illusion of the dream while simultaneously dreaming everything in the dream into existence. This experience leads to direct insight into the nature of the illusion that binds us to *samsara*. This experience can wake us up for good.

Onwards into the Dream

If you sleep, you dream, and if you dream, you can lucid dream. Whether you sleep in the park or the palace, lucid dreaming is available to you. It is your birthright. Unrestricted by censorship or state control, limited only by your relationship with your own inner state, lucid dreaming is a taste of true freedom.

If properly cultivated, lucid dreaming training may become one of the greatest advancements in psychological self-development that the 21st century has seen. Its potential is huge and yet at present we are barely scratching the surface. I believe that lucid dreaming (or at least awareness of how sleep and dreaming can be used for psycho-spiritual development) could become part of children's education in much the same way that mindfulness has been introduced into some British schools today. I envisage a time when we may have 'lucid dreaming therapists' who will use the medium of the lucid dream to help their clients commune with aspects of their unconscious. Just as we might have a 4 p.m. appointment with our hypnotherapist, so we might have a 4 a.m. appointment with our lucid dreaming therapist, who will be ready to guide us into sleep and advise us on what to do in our next lucid dream.

The parallels with hypnosis being accepted as a therapeutic treatment are quite relevant. The psychological benefits of hypnosis were known about for hundreds of years, but it wasn't until the 1950s that the American and British Medical Associations approved hypnotherapy as an orthodox treatment. It is also likely to take time for the therapeutic benefits of lucid dreaming to be validated by Western medical science, but eventually it will happen. When it does happen, as a reader of this book you will be able to count yourself as a frontier explorer, a pioneer who was willing to engage the magical potential of lucidity before the majority.

Lucid dreaming is a movement, and you are now part of it. Come and train with me at a workshop or retreat. Come and join the next Lucid Dream Facilitator training to learn how to offer lucid dreaming to your clients. This is just the beginning.

If there ever comes a time when a bizarre occurrence on a London tube train is met with a carriage full of people flipping their hands as a reality check, or a time when 'lucid dreaming' is prescribed by doctors, we will know that this movement has made it into the mindstream of the mainstream. And I want it to become mainstream. It's not the fashionable preserve of some spiritual élite, it's one of the most accessible mind-training methods in existence, and it requires nothing more than sleep to practise it. Don't keep lucid dreaming to yourself – share it with others and you will share a gift more precious than any object, because you will share a potential that, if realized, may change their lives forever.

The Buddhist master Dilgo Khyentse Rinpoche once said, 'The outer universe – the earth, stones, mountains, rocks, and cliffs – seems to be permanent and stable, like the city built of concrete. In fact, there is nothing solid to it at all; it is nothing but a city of dreams.'[1] Into this city of dreams we are born over and over again, unaware of the matrix of illusion that creates it. Lucid dreaming shows us how to make friends with illusion while we sleep, so that we can be free from illusion while we're awake.

To lucid dream is to peep behind the magician's curtain. This doesn't spoil the magic, though. Once we see how the illusion works, we still enjoy the show, but we watch less with awe and more with laughter. Through lucid dreaming, we learn how to wake up and smile at the magic.

So, let us move forward together, as dreamers in the same dream, onwards, towards dreams of awakening...

APPENDIX I
MINDFULNESS MEDITATION

There are many different types of meditation available, and if you already have a practice that works for you, then feel free to stick to that. The following practice is based upon what I was taught by Rob Nairn, and a similar practice is still being taught by the organization he founded, the Mindfulness Association. Mindfulness has so many benefits for both our waking and dreaming lives that it is well worth doing regularly, whether sitting or walking.

Sitting Meditation

The following practice might take between 20 and 30 minutes, but you can extend it for as long as you like, spending the greater portion of it in the 'resting' and 'resting with support' stages.

. . . .

Let's Do Nothing!

Sit on a hard-backed chair or cross-legged on a cushion on the floor. Make sure that you're comfortable and have your back straight.*

---

* Western science thinks that sitting up straight is good for you, too. Professor Richard Wiseman cites scientific studies that show that sitting with a straight back leads to an increase in both happiness and mathematical ability.[1]

First, settle your mind by focusing in a very relaxed way on your breath. Breathe in a little more deeply than normal and then gently release the breath.

You might like to keep your in- and out-breaths equal in length, breathing in to a count of three or four and breathing out to a count of three or four.

If possible, keep your eyes open, but if you would rather close them, that's fine too.

When you have thoughts, just let them go freely, without attempting to reject or engage them. Simply leave them alone and guide your focus back to the breathing and counting.

After a few minutes, begin to focus a little more on the out-breath and drop the counting. Notice that as you release the out-breath, your body relaxes a little. This is how you settle your mind.

Now ground your mind in your body by dropping any regulation of breath* and bringing your focus to your body. Simply become aware of all the bodily sensations you are experiencing. That's all.

You might find that a systematic scanning of your body works well for this. To do this, scan your body quite slowly, starting from your feet and ending at your head, then return to your feet and do it again.

Alternatively, you might choose to simply sit and allow your bodily sensations to command your attention as they arise. Becoming aware of the contact points of your body on the floor or seat and noticing any points of bodily tension or relaxation works well.

Become aware of how your body is supported by the ground beneath you. Feel the weight of your body creating pressure where you're sitting.

---

* The only time you regulate your breath and count is during the settling stage. By lightly regulating your breath then, you are working with the respiratory system and coming into an awareness of a henceforth automatic process.

Relax into the unconditional support of the ground. Be aware of how gravity roots you.

Once you've scanned your body or allowed your attention to be aware of particular sensations, become aware of your whole body as it sits in space. Hold your entire body within your awareness.

Allow yourself to experience how your body exists in space and is surrounded by space. This is how you ground your mind in your body.

Once you have grounded your mind in your body for about five to ten minutes, move on to resting. Rest your mind by letting go of any sense of focus on your body or breath. Simply rest. Don't try to meditate, just sit there. Give up any idea of trying to do anything. Simply be aware and in touch with whatever comes to you with a panoramic awareness.

The point of resting is to allow your mind to relax deeply and to let go of any sense of striving, struggling or trying to achieve. It isn't directed in any way, but involves simply being in the moment.

See if you can rest in this way for two or three minutes at first. This is the highest form of meditation – a flash of the mind's natural unlimited openness. Because our minds are very unsettled, we usually find this state very elusive. However, here we are momentarily tasting this freedom, so we can sense its possibility.

When you notice that your mind is becoming involved with thoughts (which might happen after just a few seconds), you can move on to resting with sound as the support.

There are many mindfulness supports that you can use, such as your breath or bodily sensations, but I've found that sound is a particularly accessible support for most people.

For sound to become the support for your mindfulness, simply focus your attention on any and all of the sounds that you can hear. Allow sound to anchor your awareness in the present moment.

Don't reject or engage with any of the sounds you can hear, just open up to whatever sounds are naturally present around you: cars outside, footsteps in the next room, the rustling of your clothes, even your own heartbeat.

Try to hear rather than listen. Listening is often goal-driven and preferential, whereas hearing is more relaxed and open. Just hear and be aware of sound.

Whenever you drift away into thought and realize *Oh, I am thinking!*, just very gently, with kind patience and without irritation, return your attention to your sound support. Remind yourself that there is nothing wrong, your distracted mind is giving you an opportunity to exercise your muscle of mindfulness, that's all.

Just sit there, knowing (and hearing) what is happening while it is happening, and each time you drift off, gently bring your mind back to the awareness of sound. Spend about 10 to 15 minutes resting your mind like this, with sound as the support.

Top Tips for Sitting Meditation

* This practice can be done at any time of day or night, but if you can, do it just before bed – all the better for lucid dreaming. The great dream yogi Tenzin Wangyal Rinpoche says that there is the potential for 'the entire night to be a deep meditation, but it requires a preparation of about 20 minutes'.[2] So, be sure to brush your teeth, let the dog out or do whatever needs to be done before you start your bedtime mindfulness session.

* Never try to stop your thoughts when you meditate. Although you don't want to engage 'thinking' as such, thoughts will always be part of your mind, just as waves are part of the sea. They

aren't something that needs to be subdued, 'rather they are direct expressions of mind's pure, luminous nature'.[3]

• You might like to infuse your meditation with the intention to gain lucidity within your dreams by thinking before you start, *As I train in my capacity for mindful awareness, may I also train in my capacity for lucidity, for the benefit of all beings.** By doing this, you are saturating your meditative mind with the intention to gain awareness within your dreams.

• Likewise, at the end of your session, be sure to dedicate the beneficial energy that you will naturally have generated to being more mindfully aware in both your waking life and dreams to the benefit of all beings.

• Then, once you get up from your seat or cushion, try to maintain the flavour of the meditation and the intention to be more mindfully aware as you continue with your day or prepare for sleep.

Walking Meditation

For those readers who are kinaesthetic learners, it's worth noting that meditation doesn't have to involve sitting still. In my early twenties I spent many years working in the professional breakdance scene and I would often see the one-pointed concentration and mindful awareness of meditation being displayed by the b-boys as they spun on their heads. Don't worry, I'm not going to suggest that

---

* It has been scientifically proven that working for the benefit of others also benefits you. When we help others, the two ancient happiness regions of the brain (the *caudate nucleus* and the *nucleus accumbens*) are stimulated, making us feel happy.

you all start breakdancing, but those of you who do like to move might like to try walking meditation.*

Walking meditation is a simple but profound practice** and just as easy to learn as sitting meditation. There are many different ways to do it, but here's one of my favourites:

....

Let's Walk!

Choose a straight path or flat area about 15 to 20 steps long and simply walk mindfully and slowly from one end of it to the other, turn around and walk back.

As you walk, centre your gaze at a 45-degree angle in front of you (with your eyes open of course!) and direct your attention to your feet. Focus on the sensation of your feet connecting with the ground.

Just as you use sound as your support in mindfulness meditation, here you use the sensations in your feet and body as you walk as your support.

Be fully aware of every feeling that arises from walking. Really enter into the feeling of taking each step – your foot lifting, passing through space and then making contact with the ground as you move forward.

Let your posture be upright but relaxed. Let your hands hang by your side or clasp them gently in front of you. See if you can avoid lapsing into a stroll or amble and can maintain full awareness of every movement you make.

---

* For something somewhere between the two, I would recommend trying the wonderful combination of dance, movement and meditation that the School of Movement Medicine offers.

** When we walk, we usually do so with some goal in mind, either to get from A to B or for exercise. Walking meditation, however, has no goal. This allows our overused goal-orientation system some well-needed rest.

Experiment with pace; some people like waking really slowly, others at a faster pace, but don't rush, take your time. You might like to regulate your breathing in time with each step, but take it nice and slow.

As you walk, try to open up your senses to the whole experience of walking. While maintaining a primary focus on the sensations of your feet, you can also have a broad panoramic awareness of the environment in which you are walking.

Try to practise for 10 or 15 minutes when you first begin and then gradually increase your practice time as you wish.

Charlie says

'I love walking meditation. It's such a great way to integrate mindfulness into your everyday life, because after you've been practising it for a while, it seeps naturally into your everyday walking habits. You find yourself lightly guiding your breath to the rhythm of your footsteps as you walk to the shops. It even changes the way you dance and the way you run!'

APPENDIX II
A SELECTION OF LUCID DREAMS AND CLARITY DREAMS

Here I'm presenting a selection of some of the most interesting lucid dreams and clarity dreams that I've experienced over the past 20 years or so. There's even the odd out-of-body experience thrown in there, too. They've been transcribed exactly as written in my dream diaries, but I've taken the liberty of editing out any insignificant or boring bits.

The 'Prep' parts are lists of the techniques, causes and conditions that may have led to that particular lucid dream. Making these lists is a good habit to get into, because it allows you to see any patterns that emerge and to analyse which techniques work best for you.

Dream 1: Amazing Clarity Dream with Dilgo Khyentse Rinpoche
May 2003

Although this was a clarity dream rather than an actual lucid dream, it is without doubt one of the most important dreams I have ever had.

I never met Dilgo Khyentse Rinpoche – he died in 1991 – and although I knew that this dream was special, it has taken years of dream yoga practice for me to truly appreciate just how important it was for me. Whether it was just an egotistical projection from my 19-year-old mind or whether it really was my inner guru who spoke to me, I still don't know, and perhaps it doesn't really matter, because this dream has served as a source of beneficial inspiration for me ever since.

After the Sogyal Rinpoche Easter retreat I prayed to meet Dilgo Khyentse Rinpoche in my next dream and that's exactly what happened.

In the dream there was a big fight as well as some sort of sexual aspect and then Dilgo Khyentse Rinpoche appeared.

He looked at me with a sort of loving disapproval, like a loving mother who's caught a child being naughty, as if he was a bit disappointed at having been invoked in such a violent dream, but he was still quite happy looking. I tried to reassure him by saying, 'You are a great master and I won't confuse the man with the lama,' and then he smiled and replied, 'For only two lifetimes I have been calling you, and now you have heard. You have good potential.'

I woke up crying.

Dream 2: Lucid Meditation
24 July 2003

This was the first time that I tried meditating in a lucid dream. I was only 19 and didn't really know what I was doing, but nonetheless it was a hugely impactful experience.

I got lucid and began to fly around the dreamscape. I remembered my current dream plan: to try to meditate in a lucid dream!

I flew up to the top of a very tall pillar and got into meditation posture. I was so excited. I'd wanted to try meditating in a lucid dream for ages, but always seemed to get involved in something else (sex, usually!) before I could.

As I sat on top of the pillar, I started to watch my breath and to meditate. Within seconds, my mind began to blow. I entered into an experience of bliss (or what I think bliss is like!) followed by an intense rushing feeling. I thought my brain was going to explode; it was like normal meditation × 1,000!

Then I heard the voice of my friend Carlos, like a sports commentator, saying, 'The meditation is becoming too powerful to comprehend,' which worried me a bit, so I managed to bring myself back to my dream body and out of the meditation.

I then flew down from the pillar into a town that seemed to be somewhere in Tibet or Nepal. When the people in the town looked at me, they either stared in shock or they covered their eyes. Their reaction scared me a bit, so I woke up.

I lay in bed buzzing. That was so cool! I hadn't prepared myself for something as intense as that. Next time I'm gonna recite mantras and see if I can invoke buddhas.

Dream 3: Lucid Self-Manifestation as Chenrezig
28 February 2007

This was a pivotal dream for me. As I look back over almost 25 years of my dream journals, it's fascinating to see how certain lucid dreams have become real milestones for me. This one was the first time that I successfully practised real dream yoga based on the oral instructions of a dream yoga master.

I became spontaneously lucid and remembered the instructions that Lama Yeshe Rinpoche had given me two weeks before about taking on the form of Chenrezig buddha in a lucid dream. So, with full lucidity, I said the mantra of Chenrezig, 'Om mani pemé hung,' and then looked down expectantly to see if I had taken on the form of Chenrezig, but I hadn't.

The lucidity was crystal-clear, though. I was flying high up above the world, reciting the Om mani pemé hung mantra and consciously dedicating it to the wellbeing of all the people below, and it felt very powerful.

I then landed back on the ground and worked through the visualization of the four-armed form of Chenrezig point by point. Strangely, I could remember exactly where each arm was positioned and what each arm held – something I'm rubbish at in waking life! Although I couldn't see it because my eyes were closed during the visualization, I could feel that I was physically taking on the form of Chenrezig. Again I flew up into the sky and recited the Mani mantra for the benefit of all beings, but this time I was in the actual form of the four-armed Chenrezig.

Suddenly I felt the presence of doom or pure darkness mocking me and challenging me. I was still flying and reciting the Om mani pemé hung mantra, but this time incredibly quickly, far more quickly than I could ever recite it in real life. Quicker and quicker and quicker it went, until the intensity started to make the lucidity slip and the dreamscape completely transformed.

I was now in a totally new dreamscape in the body of a small child walking in a procession of adults, still 100 per cent lucid. One of the adults in the procession in front of me turned around and smiled at me. As he turned, I saw that it was Lama Yeshe!

Dream 4: Teachings from Lama Yeshe Rinpoche
31 December 2007

I dreamed that I had just fallen off a cliff and the sense of falling became a lucidity trigger and I realized that I was dreaming. I managed to hover in mid-air before I hit the ground. With full lucidity, I flew into a modern-looking Moroccan-style living room. I thought, I must get teachings from Lama Yeshe, and willed him to appear.

Instantly a human form appeared on the sofa in front of me. It looked plain-faced, like a blank canvas of a human form. I prayed for Lama Yeshe to enter this form and soon he stated to appear within it. Eventually the entire form transformed into Lama Yeshe. There he was, sitting on the sofa in front of me, clear as day, looking totally realistic.

I said to him, 'Lama Yeshe, what meditation practices should I do?'

He confidently replied, 'Given that you have one and a half hours [a day?], 45 minutes for dream practice and 45 minutes for waking practice, you should do 45 minutes waking practice many times and then you will gain control over the six channels.'

As he spoke, he looked into a golden bowl full of dark liquid that was on a coffee table in front of him, and golden images formed on the surface of the liquid, illustrating what he was telling me. I saw an Eye of Buddha symbol and an African mask being traced in gold on the surface of the liquid.

Still fully lucid, I continued to receive teachings from Lama Yeshe, but when I asked him to explain more, he vanished into thin air like a ghost in a movie.

I woke myself up and wrote this all down. Was it really him or just a projection of my own inner guru archetype? Not sure, but in the *waking state the teachings still seem valid, so I guess that's all that matters.*

Dream 5: Shadow Integration
8 January 2008

This was one of the first times that I ever consciously integrated my shadow within a lucid dream and it's the dream that I referenced in my 2011 TED talk. This was also the first time I consciously hugged a shadow aspect and I have been hugging them ever since!

After a false awakening I dreamed that I was being cornered in a dark outside car park by three menacing figures, two men and one woman. They were radiating malicious intent and the fear made me become lucid.

I called out, 'Dream! This is all a dream!'

They answered, 'So what? You're still dreaming!'

I was getting scared now, so I yelled, 'It's a dream, so I can control it! Stop, stop!' but they didn't stop, they just seemed to coalesce into one big three-headed demon.

They said, 'You can't control this!' and closed in on me, laughing at my fear.

Then, just before I was going to attack them in self-defence, I remembered what Rob Nairn had told me about dealing with the shadow. He had said that instead of fighting it in my dreams, I should embrace it and talk to it.

I called out loud, 'Shadow, my shadow!' and then wrapped my arms round the three-headed demon.

I could feel it struggling within my embrace and then a heavy metal soundtrack suddenly started playing, with the repeated vocal refrain: 'This is how you become five again. This is how you become shadow, shadow.'

As the music played, I dissolved into a green triangle of light and then the entire dreamscape, including the shadow aspects, dissolved too. It felt as though I was regressing back into the past, or back into the void, where I would meet the source of my shadow.

The next thing I knew, the three-headed shadow aspect had transformed, through my embrace, into me. I was standing in front of a direct carbon copy of myself – facing my own true self. This was the source of my shadow – not a demon, but me, of course.

Prep

Had just read Rob Nairn's letter asking me to teach lucid dreaming sometime in the future – very exciting! Had jetlag due to a flight back from India = REM rebound. Had also watched *Dawn of the Dead* = nightmares.

Dream 6: Shadow Integration Lucid Dream
10 March 2009

I dreamed that I was walking along a street with a friend. I turned to him and said, 'This feels like a dream, doesn't it? I'd better check, just in case it actually is a dream.'

I then proceeded to do a hand reality check, my hand changed and I became lucid. I was so surprised that I felt I needed to do an extra check just to be sure, so I looked at my hand and willed it to get smaller, which it did. I then willed it to get bigger, which it did.

Then I walked off the street and into a nearby room, which had about four or five different people in it. One of them looked quite scary. Knowing that all of these people were personifications of my psyche, I went around the room hugging each one of them as per usual. When I got to the scary-looking one (a big fat man dressed in a kind of police uniform), he seemed very aggressive and it dawned on me that he was a full-on shadow aspect. As I went to hug him, he bit me hard on my neck and whispered hateful stuff in my ear. His bite really hurt me and I had a flash of anger before I regained my composure and realized that this was all a dream and that he was my shadow, the very essence of my repressed capacity for violence and wrath, and so to try to fight him with anger was pure folly.

Then the shadow aspect spoke, saying, 'You will never be able to stop me biting – I am the essence of violence! Violence is my nature!'

I was scared, but I realized that I had to embrace him. I couldn't hug him, so I would have to try something new. I grabbed him and wrestled him to the floor. Then I kneeled over him and began literally to inhale him, to breathe in the essence of this darkness, to integrate this energy that I had repressed. I breathed in all the denied anger and disowned power that he contained.

As I did this, he literally began to dissolve in front of my very eyes. It was still quite scary because I could actually feel the dark energy that he embodied entering me, but I knew that the shadow couldn't hurt me if my motivation was to integrate it.

As I continued to breathe in the shadow's essence, I repeated out loud, 'I am integrated, I am balanced, I am joy, love and equanimity. I am integrated, I am balanced, I am joy, love and equanimity,' and the shadow continued to shrink and dissolve into the vapour that I was inhaling.

Once the shadow had totally dissolved, I stood up and said, in a low, wrathful voice, 'That was a good thing. Now I can be fully integrated.'

Then I woke up.

Prep

Fell asleep at about midnight doing the 'I. Am I dreaming? 2. Am I dreaming?' FAC technique. Also briefly prayed to Guru Rinpoche for a lucid dream.

Dream 7: 'What is the Essence of All Knowledge?'
9 May 2009

I dreamed that I was at a big theatre-type venue, doing a gig with my old band. After the gig, I was doing gravity-defying aerial acrobatics around the venue. The jumping up and down seemed to stimulate my lucid awareness [somatic sensation often leads to lucidity] and soon I was fully lucid.

I remembered my dream plan and put it into action. I called out to the dream: 'What is the essence of all knowledge?'

Instantly a huge game-show-style computer screen manifested in front of me with the question written across it in big digital lettering. The letters were so big that I could read them easily without them blurring. Three dots appeared after the question mark, indicating that I was about to receive the answer.

I tried hard to keep my excitement under control, but it was really difficult! Then the answer finally manifested. The computer screen read: 'The essence of all knowledge is?... Obtainable through lucid dreaming'!

I literally laughed out loud within the dream as I thought, At least my unconscious has a sense of humour!

Then I woke up.

Once awake, I opened to the possibility that maybe the answer wasn't such a joke after all. Maybe the essence of all knowledge is obtainable through lucid dreaming?

Prep

Listened to a Lama Surya Das audiobook while I fell asleep, plus I had a little bit of REM rebound from the night before. I did the FAC technique. Also, I went to sleep on a light meal and had been thinking about how heartbreak could be good for lucid dreams.

Dream 8: Meeting my Subconscious Mind
13 May 2009

This was one of those rare lucid dreams in which the healing is so deep that you can actually feel it physically the next day. A deep underlying happiness and contentment lasted for the entire day that followed, and I'm not sure it has ever completely faded.

I was in a large open-plan office space which was in a basement. There were people milling about as if some sort of 'Ideal Home Show' exhibition had finished a few hours before. I heard a man telling his son, 'Make a living! You just need to make a living!' and I felt annoyed with him for giving his son such limiting advice. For some reason I decided to do some cartwheels around the space to show the boy how he could free his thinking. The movement seemed to tip me over into lucidity and I realized that I was dreaming.

After doing a hand reality check, I became fully lucid. I tried to remember the lucid dream plan I had made, but I couldn't seem to access my memory. Eventually, after a few seconds I remembered my dream plan: to meet my subconscious mind.

Instantly the dream plan became engaged, as all the dream characters disappeared.

Just then a plain-looking woman in her early thirties appeared out of nowhere holding a clipboard. Instinctively I knew that she was something to do with this dream plan, so I went up to her and said, 'Are you my subconscious?'

She replied, 'Yes, I am.'

I felt shocked – I hadn't actually been expecting her to say yes. I asked her again, 'So, you're my subconscious mind?'

Again she said in a matter-of-fact way, 'Yes, that's right.'

I was lost for words, but eventually I got my head together and said, 'Oh, OK. Great. Well… how am I?'

She replied, 'You're good. You're fine, really.'

I then felt an overwhelming desire to confess to her and to apologize to her for all that I'd put us though. So I began admitting to all the bad things I'd done in my life and apologizing about all the people I'd wronged. There was no guilt, though – it felt good. It was an experience of real catharsis, and once I'd finished, the woman smiled and said, 'It's alright. I know you're working on that.' She was so accepting of me and not angry or judgemental.

It felt that there was nothing left to be said, so I hugged her and I woke up crying with happiness. Lying in my bed, I felt very different. Something had shifted.

Prep

Taught the MILD technique that evening and then practised MILD after 7.15 a.m. wake-up.

Dream 9: Buddha Nature Lucid!
11 January 2010

I dreamed that I threw a dog's paw through a first-storey apartment window, an act so bizarre that I habitually did a reality check: I tried to read some text on a sign in the courtyard of the apartment block, but it was all jumbled and so I knew I was dreaming.

Now fully lucid, I flew up into the overcast evening sky and engaged my current dream plan by calling out to the sky, 'I want to meet my Buddha nature. Show me my Buddha nature!'

Then I looked down at the ground, expecting to see a monk or wise man or some other archetypal representation of my Buddha nature.

Nobody appeared, but suddenly the cloudy evening sky was illuminated by a bright orange glow, as if the sun had just risen to its highest point.

'What about my Buddha nature? I want to meet my Buddha nature!' I complained, until it clicked: I was meeting my Buddha nature! This was it! My Buddha nature was illumination, bright light in an evening sky, sunlight from behind the clouds, a luminous glow!

I was then joined by two or three other people and we flew over the desert terrain towards the sun before I woke up, feeling totally blissed out.

Prep

Fell asleep after 6 a.m. wake-up reciting the script of the dream plan: 'In my next lucid dream I meet my Buddha nature.' I had also been to teachings on Buddha nature that evening and was sleeping in the spare room at Mum's house (different bed = good for lucidity).

Dream 10: Lama Yeshe Clarity Dream
19 January 2010

I was at some sort of boatyard and had broken my leg and was losing a lot of blood. Even so, I felt fearless and was determined not to die and to get myself to safety. I was dragging myself along wooden decking to the edge of the boatyard, where there was a ferry waiting to take me to the other side of the harbour and to safety.

Then suddenly I saw Lama Yeshe Rinpoche over by the ferry crossing, just standing there waiting happily. I didn't want to cause a fuss or disturb him, so I simply greeted him warmly as I hauled myself still bleeding onto the ferry boat.

Once I was aboard, Lama Yeshe asked me, 'Where are you going?'

I replied, 'I've broken my leg, lama, and I need to get to the other side or I might die.'

He cheerfully acknowledged my situation by saying, 'Oh, I see! Yes, OK then,' as I floated off on the ferry boat. Then he smiled broadly and called out to me, 'Don't worry, I will bring you over. It will happen subtly at first and there won't be lots of chances, but I will bring you over.'

Dream 11: Career Path Lucidity
27 August 2010

After years of doubt over whether I was qualified to teach dream work, and recurring dreams reflecting that doubt, I finally managed to become lucid and ask the Dreamer what they thought I should do. Their answer set me on the path of a whole new career.

I dreamed that I was watching a big house fill up with water and burst under the pressure. I watched the doors and windows explode outwards, with water gushing out and forming a tsunami that rushed out onto the street on which I stood! After an initial flash of fear, I thought to myself, I reckon I can surf this wave – I'm gonna be alright! and I bodysurfed the tsunami as it swept me off my feet.

The fear seemed to boost my awareness and I soon became fully lucid. I realized within the dream that the house bursting under pressure was symbolic of the doubt that I had been feeling. So then I thought that this would be the perfect opportunity to ask my higher self/unconscious mind for some advice about this.

After a couple of reality checks to solidify the lucidity, I called out to the sky, 'How can I be of most benefit? Should I do the lucid dreaming or should I do THROWDOWN [the hip-hop group that I used to run]?'

In an instant the entire dreamscape dissolved into a drinks party in the living room of a small house. The room was full of people standing around chatting and I realized beyond doubt that each person in the room was an aspect of my own psyche who would have an answer to my question.

I spotted a man in white robes who looked like a cross between a Buddhist monk and a vicar (a personification of my spiritual side?)

and I went up to him and asked, 'What should I do with my life? Should I teach lucid dreaming or do THROWDOWN?'

He replied with great sincerity and clasped his hands in prayer, saying, 'Of course you must do the lucid dream teaching. That is of most benefit.'

Then I saw a teenager standing in the corner of the room, knocking back shots (a personification of my hedonistic side?) and I went up to him and asked the same question. His reply was to offer me a shot of vodka and yell, 'THROWDOWN rocks, man!'

Still with full lucidity and chuckling to myself about how my unconscious was choosing to portray my wild side, I then went and asked a pretty neutral-looking woman and a 30-something man what they thought I should do with my life, and they both said that I should do the lucid dream teaching too.

Satisfied that I had got a balanced opinion from these aspects of my own psyche, I walked out of the house and found myself on an urban street at dusk. Why hadn't I woken up yet? I usually wake up after I've been given the punchline/teaching.

As I walked away from the house, I was thinking about how supportive my unconscious had been. Then I suddenly felt the urge to turn round and look back at the house. I did and I saw all the dream characters that I had just been talking to huddled around the window, watching me walk away. When they saw me turn round, they all started smiling and waving. It was so unexpected!

I felt as though my heart would burst with joy and I yelled out, 'Unconscious, subconscious, conscious mind, I love you all! Thank you so much for everything!'

Then the dream characters started calling out, 'Good luck, Charlie! We love you, too!'

I woke up because of the wetness of tears on my pillow. I was crying with happiness. Any doubt over what I should do with my life was gone. I felt an unshakable confidence and faith.

I want to teach lucid dreaming and I want to help people.

Dream 12: Teachings on Pain and Suffering
12 November 2010

I became lucid gradually in a dream in which I was on the New Year's Eve retreat with Tim Freke, a Gnostic scholar. He said, 'You now know that you are dreaming and I will guide you through the lucid dream.' This comment brought me to full lucidity, as I realized that I was actually already lucid and this was all a dream!

Then, without warning, Tim produced a huge flaming log of wood and smashed it over my back as I stood next to him in front of the group. The burning embers shattered and poured down my back and onto the floor around my feet. I felt the intense pain of the burning coals singeing my skin and scorching my back. I realized that this must be some sort of upright 'fire-walking' demonstration. Tim said it was 'a teaching about the difference between pain and suffering'.

The pain felt so real, but as the group stood around me, watching the burning embers scorch my skin, Tim looked at me with a kind face and smiled. With that smile, I realized what this demonstration was about. I felt pain because I'd had a burning log smashed over my back, but I felt no suffering because I knew that this was all a dream. I was fully aware that the pain was merely a projection of my own mind and that suffering was caused by aversion to pain, not by pain itself.

In the lucid dream I could feel pain and yet I wasn't suffering – this was what Tim was teaching me. He was explaining this to the group as I stood there and they all seemed to understand it.

I also realized that pain in the waking state was also illusory and that so much of our suffering was self-inflicted, due to our powerful rejection of all pain and discomfort.

Once the demonstration was over, Tim asked me to help 'polish and clean everybody's light bulbs' and we proceeded to go down the line of people polishing their light bulbs, which seemed somehow to be an outward expression of their consciousness.

Prep

Woke at 11.58 p.m. after going to bed at 10.10 p.m. and falling asleep reciting, 'I want to recognize my dreams and realize the awareness that lies beyond my projections.' I also spent a few hours reading Tim's book (*The Laughing Jesus* by Timothy Freke and Peter Gandy).

Dream 13: One Hundred-Syllable Mantra Lucid Dream
23 December 2010

This was one of the most memorable lucid dreams I have ever had. It went on for so long, contained so many different elements – everything from mantra recitation to shadow integration – and had such a funny musical-theatre ending that it still makes me laugh!

I dreamed that I was discussing with a nun how crazy it was that I might be in a dream and that at one point I might wake up in a bed in a future world and find that everything had been a dream. Then I realized that I was actually dreaming right then!

I looked around and saw that I was in a huge empty hall, as big as a warehouse. I did hand reality checks, got fully lucid and engaged my current dream plan of chanting the 100-syllable purification mantra within the lucid dream.

As I began to chant, I could feel a huge movement of energy and soon I saw loads of people rushing towards me from each end of the huge space. Suddenly I felt a flash of fear and thought, Oh God, I'm chanting a purification mantra, so I'm going to invoke loads of shadow aspects! But then, as they came closer, I saw that they were in fact all maroon-robed monks and nuns. There were hundreds of them, all flocking into the hall, beckoned by the mantra. Within a few seconds, they had assembled and sat down in rows and a chant master had appeared on a fully kitted-out stage with musicians playing the tune of the chant and they were all chanting along with me in unison! All these projections of my own mind chanting together!

I saw that Lama Yeshe Rinpoche had appeared, too, and was sitting on a high throne facing the stage. Still totally lucid, I went over to him and asked if I could sit in the empty space next to him. He seemed to be in deep meditation, but nodded in affirmation. So there I sat, on the right-hand side of Lama Yeshe, with hundreds of Tibetan monks and nuns all chanting the 100-syllable mantra together within the lucid dream! Amazing!

Soon after this, I heard more people arriving, not monks and nuns, but projections of everyday people, and some of my shadow aspects (sexualized/angry-looking people), who had heard the call of the purification mantra, too, but, unlike the monks and nuns, weren't there to sit quietly! The shadow aspects were there for trouble!

I turned round and started to chant at the shadow aspects directly, which seemed to rile them even more. They didn't like my attempt to purify them! So I waded into the crowd of shadow aspects and started hugging them and integrating them through hugs and telling them that I loved them. I just kept going up to the most offensive-looking ones and kissing them with love.

Then I became super-lucid as I remembered that in lucid dreams we are one with everything, even with inanimate objects. I had knocked over a chair during a fracas with a shadow aspect, so I went and picked it up and actually started hugging and kissing it! I was ecstatic in the knowledge that I was inside my own head and that the more love and appreciation that I could show to each and every thing, the more loving and appreciative my mind would become in waking life!

Throughout all this, the monks and nuns had continued to chant the 100-syllable mantra and so I decided to make my way up to the stage, where the chant master and musicians were leading the chant. When I got up on stage, they stopped the music and chanting and I found myself facing the audience of about 500 monks and nuns and a few hundred everyday dream characters and shadow aspects. I saw a dream character who I knew was a representation of a deeply beneficial part of my unconscious and I wanted him to get up on stage so that I could thank him. As I took the mic, the band started up as if they wanted me to sing, and the crowd was calling for a song too!

Still lucid and totally aware that this was all a dream, I started to sing from my heart, 'I love you all! I really do! I love you all! I love you so much!' I sang it over and over, and soon the whole room was singing it together! All these aspects of my own psyche were singing, 'I love you so much, I love you so much!' to a tune of 'Da dee da dee, da dee dee da dee'! It was so funny, but so beautiful too that my unconscious mind became an expression of pure love! I was crying and calling out over the singing, 'Make me kinder! Make me more loving! Make me more beneficial! I love you all! Thank you so much!'

I woke up crying with joy, totally blissful.

Prep

Kickboxing energy drink led to restless sleep, read Théun Mares' Toltec book, went to bed on an empty stomach, lunar eclipse last night. Sleeping on the sofa at Mum's place. Been doing a lot more Vajrasattva purification practice in the past two weeks.

Dream 14: Huge Lucid Dream with Walking Through Walls and Entry into the Void!
22 April 2011

After two false awakenings, I became fully lucid. My lucidity has been so slack recently that I really wanted to make this a nice long LD to get back on track. I called out, 'Stabilize lucidity! The lucidity is deep and stable!' and my lucid awareness deepened.

The dreamscape was a big, airy, high-ceilinged shopping mall full of people walking around shopping. As I walked through the mall, I decided to do some wall-walking. I went up to a dark granite stone wall which formed part of a shop front, reminded myself, I'm dreaming so I can stick my hand through this wall, then stuck my hand into it up to my elbow.

I took time to really experience how it felt. It was as if my arm was in a vat of partially solidified concrete. It was a thick viscous liquid rock and when I grasped at it I could feel the detail of the coarse grains of granite through my fingertips. I even managed to pull a handful of the liquid rock out of the wall. I watched as it collected like mercury in the palm of my hand and began to harden before my very eyes.

I then set the intention that the wall would now be solid and I tapped on it and it was kind of solid, like liquid with a hard film over it.

I looked around, saw another wall that formed part of a different shop and decided run through it. I set the intention that on the other side of the wall I would find the dazzling darkness of the void. As I ran through the wall, I called out, 'Clear light now! For the benefit of all beings, clear light now!'

On the other side of the wall I found myself floating in the vast deep-space blackness of the void. From within the blackness, huge archetypal images of golden light manifested. Snakes, dragons and ancient-looking creatures were traced in gold across the blackness. They began flicking up into my field of vision in very quick succession and it felt like some sort of download of information from the collective mind into my mind. It soon became too intense and I woke up.

Prep

Went to sleep after 20 minutes of meditation on the reversed red Tibetan syllable 'ah' in the throat chakra. Then fell asleep sounding the 'ah' sound and offering prayers for lucidity. Fifteen minutes of meditation at shrine from 5 a.m. Woke again after LD at 6.45 a.m.

Dream 15: Guru Rinpoche Self-manifestation and OBE with Lama Yeshe
21 November 2011

Before bed I set a strong intention to have a life-changing lucid dream. I was literally praying over and over, saying, 'Give me a lucid dream so powerful that it changes everything, for the benefit of all beings!' And it seems that my prayers were heard loud and clear.

Lucid dream after 4.30 a.m. wake-up. Using FAC method, I went straight into a dream and looked at my hands once lucid. I then engaged my dream plan of calling out the long invocation mantra of Guru Rinpoche. I called it out three times so loudly I thought I might have even been calling out in my sleep, and then I began levitating into the air and transforming into Guru Rinpoche.

It was a slow transformation into the form of Guru Rinpoche, but I actually manifested his ornaments and everything. This was full deity self-manifestation. It felt very powerful and very stable.

After this, I floated up and saw a computer screen with an outer-space screensaver on it, so I used it as a portal by climbing into it and thus into the space scene that it depicted.

Once in space, I engaged the OBE practice and called out, 'Out of body now! Lama Yeshe Rinpoche now!' and got whizzed off at great speed into the pitch-black space. I was going very fast through several layers/slices of space and it seemed as though I was passing through the very fabric of the universe.

Then suddenly I arrived in a kind of office space with little cubicles and desks, but quite big and open-plan, very solid, very OBE, not dreamlike at all.

As soon as I arrived, a big fat Black guy ran up to me and hugged me. He seemed very surprised to see me, but happy nonetheless. I then realized that it was Lama Yeshe Rinpoche!

After the initial greeting, he seemed to think that I had come at a not-so-perfect time and he politely made his excuses. It seemed that I had arrived unannounced and that although he was happy to see me, it wasn't a good time for him. Maybe it was because he was in this different form?

Prep

Ngöndro practice dedicated to 'Give me a lucid dream so powerful that it changes everything, for the benefit of all beings!' And lots of prayers and true confidence that I would get lucid. Woke at 4.30 a.m. then did FAC perfectly and prayers, including a long invocation mantra as I fell asleep with a visualization of Guru Rinpoche and Lama Yeshe in heart centre.

Dream 16: Ear-Infection Healing Dream
6 August 2012

I went surfing in New York and picked up a nasty ear infection that blocked my ear completely with wax – 'glue ear', they called it. I tried ear drops (and everything else I could think of), but they didn't seem to work, so I stopped using them. A few days later I became lucid and experienced my first direct physical manifestation of healing from within the lucid dream state.

Woke at about 4 a.m. after a very long healing lucid dream! Got lucid from the lights in the dream not working and hand reality checks. First I called out to all the dream characters, 'You are all aspects of my own psychology and I love you all!' Then I went over to a guy in a linen jacket and started touching the jacket, exploring how amazingly real it felt. I asked him what the material was and he said, 'Crosshatched brushed cotton.'

I said, 'What? I don't think I even know what that is.'

He replied, 'Maybe it's from your memory stores?'

Then I remembered my dream plan and engaged it: 'Heal my ear! Please, immune system, engage your healing power to heal me of my ear infection! Please help me to heal my glue ear! My ear is healed!'

Within the dream, I could actually hear and feel my ear being unblocked. It felt so realistic. I could hear the wax being broken up in my ear canal as if I had just put in ear drops! The sensation woke me up and I discovered that the dream had actually manifested a physical response! That's why it felt so realistic! Lying in my bed, wide awake, my ear was now unblocking and wax was streaming out of it. So gross, but so cool!

The following lucid dreams do not appear in the first edition of this book. These new ones give you an idea of the kind of things that I am currently using lucid dreaming to explore and hopefully serve to inspire you to try out some of these dream plans too.

Dream 17: Huge 'Show Me Something Important' Lucid Dream!
16 November 2020

Got lucid after flying out of a window in fear of being blown up by a bomb. As I flew, the act of flying became a trigger and I became semi-lucid and then I started singing and chanting, 'I am in a lucid dream! I am in a lucid dream!' over and over until I was fully lucid.

Without a set dream plan, I defaulted to 'Show me something important!', but when I called it out, nothing was manifesting, so I said, 'Show me something important in the space behind this wall!' just so I could be sure to get something and to give the Dreamer time to manifest something.

Then when I looked behind the wall a little boy appeared and then another. Both were disabled and wanted to show me their dancing and singing, and I played with them and felt very loving towards them. In the dream I realized that they were my disabled inner child and I felt so loving towards them.

Then, as the dream was still continuing, I tried doing the same sankalpa again and called out, 'Show me something important!' and then a 30-something white guy appeared and said that he was Time. He was the personification of the concept of time.

I was excited and thought how cool this was and so I asked him how time worked and he told me to hop on for a piggy-back ride, and when I did, he started teaching me how we are all piggy-backing on time. As he moved, I realized that he was showing me how the time–space continuum worked, because he was moving forward along a linear line and space was changing around him, a bit like when Cooper is in the tesseract in the movie Interstellar. Then he told me, 'Time is the vehicle that moves you through reality and life.'

I then thought of asking Time himself a question, as surely he would know the past, present and future, and so I whispered into his ear while still piggy-backing on him, 'How can I deal with my mum dying?' and he told me, through images and a hand-drawn diagram, that although I would encounter dead-ends and doors that wouldn't open, when that happened I should just turn around and try another door. He said, 'One door will always open for you,' as I clung to his back like a child.

This was so moving to hear that I started to cry and the tears woke me up.

Prep

A 5 a.m. wake-up with a slow descent back to sleep. A two-hour LD drop-in that evening. Gave the dream plan to a lady from the drop-in, so wanted to try it myself.

Dream 18: 'How Can I Be of Most Benefit?'
24 April 2021

Got lucid from a false awakening in which I was in my living room watching a video recording of Zia on WhatsApp saying how he had bumped his head, but actually it had been gushing blood and had congealed. Things he was saying just didn't make sense, so I started to Columbo-method the situation and soon realized that I might be dreaming, so I did a hand reality check and it morphed, so I became lucid.

Couldn't recall my dream plan so I defaulted to wall-walking and went headfirst into a painting of Quan Yin, and then I went over to the balcony and decided to ask a question to the Dreamer and called out, 'How can I be of most benefit?'

I yelled it out to the night sky and in response a huge map of the world appeared flat against the night sky. The map was created by sparkling stars or LED lights.

All the different countries were lighting up individually and then some lit up simultaneously and then every country on the whole map was lit up.

The Dreamer seemed to be telling me to 'go global' or that I should take the teachings to the entire world.

Then some words appeared in the sky expanding on this advice. It said stuff about Instagram and asking questions of people, but I can't remember what exactly. The main thing seems to be the message: 'Take it global.'

Then I looked over my balcony and there was a party going on beneath me and a nightclub or bar had been set up where the bike racks are. I then flew down onto Enid Street and was waving at people and being friendly. Then I woke up.

Prep

Excitement insomnia, lots of *chi* energy from general over-excitement about life!

Dream 19: Guru Rinpoche Clear Light Lucid Dream
15 December 2022

FAC where I saw the dream forming out of the hypnagogic and then literally was labelling the hypnagogic as it appeared, saying to myself, 'That's a computer screen, that's a desk, this is a dream,' as the images popped up, but it was too thin, it was still in the dough stage.

But then I said to myself, 'That's an office, that's a room, make it clear, it's a dream,' as if my labelling and stating what I could see was kind of cooking the dough and making it turn into the bread of the dream. It worked and I found myself in a dream, fully lucid.

Once lucid, no need to do reality checks as it was an FAC entry, so went straight into dream plan sankalpa of 'Om ah hung benza guru pema tötreng tsal benza samaya dza siddhi pala hung ah' (the long invocation mantra of Guru Rinpoche) while invoking Guru Rinpoche into the lucid dream.

I recited the mantra out loud while walking through a wall and into the blackness beyond. I did this not only to confirm the awareness of the emptiness of the dream, but also with the intention to enter the clear light of the void beyond the dream.

Then on the other side of the wall I was floating in the black void of the clear light, still saying the mantra, and I had the intention and expectation that Guru Rinpoche would appear visually from the void, but he didn't, he appeared in a form that I had never encountered before: he appeared in the form of the energy.

I started to feel huge rushes of energy from beneath me and from all angles, as if they were gusts of windhorse energy keeping me aloft as I floated in the void.

It was Guru Rinpoche, but in the form of formless energy. The rushes of energy from all angles were actually him.

Then I woke up as I lost my focus.

Prep

WBTB* after energy-body insomnia. Felt like before I have an OBE when I can feel the *chi* rushing, so I knew that I could use this energy for a lucid dream or OBE.

Dream 20: Grief Healed Through the Inner Child
30 April 2023

Dreaming I was in the Buddhist centre when I saw Lama Zangmo from behind and she had blood on her head. I thought, Why is her head bleeding? This is weird. I think I might be dreaming. And then I said to her, 'Lama, I think we're dreaming.' And she replied (just as she would have in the waking state), 'I don't think so, Charlie.'

And then a horse walked into the dream and I said, 'Come on, lama, we're definitely dreaming!'

Now fully lucid, I remembered my dream plan. I called out, 'I love you, inner child, I love you!'

As I did this, Lama Zangmo transformed into an aspect of my inner child. She maintained her form, but she started nuzzling into me like a little child or puppy dog. She had become reflection of my inner child.

Then one of the volunteers, Joelle, appeared, and I said joyfully, 'Can you bring me my inner child, please?'

---

* The 'Wake Up, Back to Bed' Method (*see page 142*)

She nodded and smiled, and then she either presented me with the inner child, or at that moment Lama Zangmo fully transformed into the inner child – I can't quite remember, but whichever it was, my inner child now appeared.

It was a blissfully joyful moment of full embrace and full sending-of-love to and hugging Little Chuck. It felt so good. So nice and warm (like when you believe in Santa), and loving and joyful.

Then I woke up crying.

Prep

Small WBTB from cycle from Chloë's at 2 a.m. after insomnia and also end of IONS* study on San Fran time zones = jet-lag dreams.

Dream 21: Lucid Clarity Dream: the Final Teaching from Rob
25 October 2023

I was at the Cape Town Samye Dzong Buddhist centre and I overheard people whispering excitedly, saying, 'Oh, is it his? Is it still there?' and I assumed they were talking about Rob Nairn's coat, which I had been given when he died, but then they said something about a prayer mat and then suddenly Rob Nairn appeared.

In a flash the scene had changed and we were all gathered around Rob, sitting at his feet while he was raised up on a chair and we were looking up at him. The mood was quite reverent and it was obvious that he was about to give a Buddhist teaching.

Then it suddenly hit me: Rob's dead, he died, I must be dreaming! And now with full lucidity and overwhelming joy, I cried out, 'Rob, oh

---

* The Institute of Noetic Sciences, California

Rob! One final teaching, please give me one final teaching! What's the most important teaching?'

He looked at me and he was smiling with such deep kindness and love in his eyes as he mouthed some words silently to me. Then he noticed that I hadn't understood what he'd said through this teaching without words, so he spoke out loud to me. He said clearly that the most important teaching was 'The Aphrodessence* of Suffering or Kindness'.

I then spoke this back to him to make sure I had it right, saying, 'The aphrodescence of suffering or kindness? Kindness! It's kindness!' and he nodded, smiling.

Then I asked him, 'Should I wake up myself up now and try to find this teaching?', to which he replied, 'No, stay.'

The emotion of the dream was becoming too intense, though. The amazement at receiving a final teaching from him after he was dead was just too much and I could feel the lucidity slipping.

I woke up.

Prep

On Delson Armstrong retreat doing hours and hours of TWIM** and metta (loving-kindness) all day, using Rob as my focus for metta, and Lama Yeshe, too. Loads of illusory body practice during the day, too, walking around the retreat telling myself constantly: 'I am asleep, I am in bed right now, sleeping. This is all a dream, I am asleep right now.'

---

*   I am aware that this isn't a real word, but it's what he said.

** Tranquil Wisdom Insight Meditation

REFERENCES

Introduction

1. Matthew Walker, *The Tim Ferriss Show Transcripts*: 'Dr Matthew Walker, All Things Sleep Continued'; https://tim.blog/2023/02/10/dr-matthew-walker-transcript/ [accessed 16 April 2024]

Chapter 1: The Basics

1. Dresler, M., *et al.*, 'Neural correlates of dream lucidity obtained from contrasting lucid versus non-lucid REM sleep: a combined EEG/fMRI case study', *Sleep* 35(7), 1 July 2012, 1,017–202

2. van Eeden, F., 'A study of dreams', *Proceedings of the Society for Psychical Research* 26, 1913, 431–61

3. Hess, G., Schredl, M., and Goritz, A.S., 'Lucid dreaming frequency and the big five personality factors', *Imagination, Cognition and Personality* 36(3), May 2016

4. Cited in Michael Katz, *Tibetan Dream Yoga*, Bodhi Tree, 2011, p.3

5. Rapport, N., 'Pleasant Dreams!', *Psychiatric Quarterly* 22, 1948, 309–17

6. Voss, U., *et al.*, 'Lucid dreaming: a state of consciousness with features of both waking and non-lucid dreaming', *Sleep* 32(9), September 2009, 1,191–200

7. Max-Planck-Gesellschaft, 'Lucid dreamers help scientists locate the seat of meta-consciousness in the brain', *ScienceDaily*, 27 July 2012; http://www.sciencedaily.com/releases/2012/07/120727095555.htm [accessed 5 September 2023]

8. Albert Einstein, Letter to Robert S. Marcus, 12 February 1950, Albert Einstein Archives, Hebrew University of Jerusalem

9. Robert Waggoner, *Lucid Dreaming*, Moment Point Press, 2009, p.17

10. *Ibid.*, p.20

11. Rob Preece, *The Psychology of Buddhist Tantra*, Snow Lion Publications, 2012, p.107

12. Lapina, N., Lysenko, V., and Burikov, A., 'Age-dependent dreaming: characteristics of secondary school pupils', *Sleep Supplement* 21, 1998, 287

13. Schredl, M., Henley-Einon, J., and Blagrove, M., 'Lucid dreaming in children: the UK library study'; Central Institute of Mental Health, Mannheim, Germany, Department of Psychology, Swansea University, United Kingdom; https://orca.cardiff.ac.uk/id/eprint/114656/1/Lucid%20dreaming%20in%20children%202012.pdf [accessed 16 April 2024]

14. Voss, U., *et al.*, 'Lucid dreaming: an age-dependent brain dissociation', *Journal of Sleep Research* 21(6), December 2012, 634–42

15. Gackenbach, J., 'Video game play and lucid dreams: implications for the development of consciousness', *Dreaming* 16(2), 2006, 96–110; https://doi.org/10.1037/1053-0797.16.2.96 [accessed 12 April 2024]

16. 'Lucid dreaming in children: the UK library study', *International Journal of Dream Research* 5, April 2012; https://www.researchgate.net/publication/277035223_Lucid_dreaming_in_children_The_UK_library_study [accessed 12 April 2024]

17. Cited in Francisco J. Varela and HH Dalai Lama, *Sleeping, Dreaming, and Dying*, Wisdom Publications, 1997, p.105

18. Cited *ibid.*, p.106

Chapter 2: The Science of Lucidity

1. Keith Hearne, *The Dream Machine*, Aquarian Press, 1990, p.12

2. Paul and Charla Devereux, *Lucid Dreaming*, Daily Grail Publishing, 2011, p.76

3. LaBerge, S., *et al.*, 'Lucid dreaming verified by volitional communication during REM sleep', *Perceptual and Motor Skills* 52, 1981, 727–32

4. Erlacher, D., *et al.*, 'Frequency of lucid dreams and lucid dream practice in German athletes', *Imagination, Cognition and Personality* 31(3), January 2011, 237–46; https://www.researchgate.net/publication/230727513_Frequency_of_Lucid_Dreams_and_Lucid_Dream_Practice_in_German_Athletes [accessed 12 April 2024]

5. Schädlich, M., and Erlacher, D., 'Practicing sports in lucid dreams: characteristics, effects, and practical implications', *Current Issues in Sport Science* 3, 2018

6. 'Can lucid dreaming make you a better athlete?' Tomorrow's World, BBC, Wellcome; https://www.youtube.com/watch?v= JQXgxMgnDQg [accessed 16 April 2024]

7. Behncke, L., 'Mental skills training for sports: a brief review', *Athletic Insight: The online journal of sport psychology* 6(1), March 2004

8. Elizabeth Quinn, 'Do visualization exercises help build strength?', www.verywellfit.com, 13 August 2020; http://sportsmedicine.about. com/od/sportspsychology/a/thinkstrong.htm [accessed 5 September 2023]

9. Robert Uhlig, 'Thinking about exercise "can beef up biceps"', *Daily Telegraph*, 22 November 2001; https://www.telegraph.co.uk/news/ worldnews/northamerica/usa/1363146/Thinking-about-exercise-can-beef-up-biceps.html [accessed 5 September 2023]

10. Filevich, E., *et al.*, 'Metacognitive mechanisms underlying lucid dreaming', *Journal of Neuroscience* 35(3), 21 January 2015, 1,082–8

11. 'Lucid dreamers have larger brain regions associated with self-reflection and metacognition', Medical Daily, 25 January 2015; https:// www.medicaldaily.com/lucid-dreaming-associated-more-pronounced-self-reflection-everyday-life-319326 [accessed 25 April 2024]

12. Bourke, P., and Shaw, H., 'Spontaneous lucid dreaming frequency and waking insight', *Dreaming* 24(2), 2014, 152–9

13. Konkoly, K.R., *et al.*, 'Real-time dialogue between experimenters and dreamers during REM sleep', *Current Biology* 31(7), 12 April 2021; https://www.sciencedirect.com/science/article/pii/S0960982221000592 [accessed 12 April 2024]

14. Freitas de Macêdo, T.C., *et al.*, 'My dream, my rules: can lucid dreaming treat nightmares?', *Frontiers in Psychology* 10, 2019; https://www.ncbi.nlm.nih.gov/pmc/articles/PMC6902039/ [accessed 12 April 2024]

Chapter 3: The Psychological Benefits of Lucid Dreaming

1. Rob Nairn in conversation with the author, 2009

2. Valerie Austin, *Self-Hypnosis*, Thorsons, 1994, p.26

3. *Ibid.*, p.27

4. Marc Barasch, *Healing Dreams*, Riverhead, 2000

5. Angela Haupt, 'Why is everyone working on their inner child?', *Time*, 6 April 2023; https://time.com/6268636/inner-child-work-healing/ [accessed 12 April 2024]

6. https://www.goodreads.com/quotes/747681-the-real-you-is-still-a-little-child-who-never [accessed 12 April 2024]

7. Sackwild, L., and Stumbrys, T., 'The healing and transformative potential of lucid dreaming for treating clinical depression', *International Journal of Dream Research* 14(2), 2021, 296–308; https://doi.org/10.11588/ijodr.2021.2.81533 [accessed 12 April 2024]

8. American Cancer Society, 'Non-medical Ways to Manage Pain; https://www.cancer.org/cancer/managing-cancer/side-effects/pain/non-medical-treatments-for-cancer-pain.html [accessed 16 April 2024]

9. Michael Katz, *Tibetan Dream Yoga*, Bodhi Tree, 2011, p.31

10. Richard Wiseman, *59 Seconds*, Pan, 2010, p.199

11. *Ibid.*, p.198

12. Ben Goldacre, 'Battling bad science', TED talk, July 2011; https://www.ted.com/talks/ben_goldacre_battling_bad_science?language=en [accessed 5 September 2023]

13. C.G. Jung, *Psychology and Religion*, 1938, in *Collected Works 11: Psychology and Religion: West and East*, Princeton University Press, 1975, p.131

14. W.B. Yeats, *Responsibilities*, Cuala Press, 1914, p.172, attributed to an 'old play'

Chapter 4: Sleeping Buddhas

1. Stephen Batchelor, 'Buddhism for this One and Only Life', the first talk of his *Tricycle* online retreat, 26 June 2010

2. Trinlay Tulku Rinpoche, 'East is West', *Tricycle* online magazine, Summer 2005, p.5

3. The *Pali Vinaya*, Oldenberg, I.295, quoted in Serenity Young, *Dreaming in the Lotus*, Wisdom Publications, 1999, p.44

4. Francisco J. Varela and HH Dalai Lama, *Sleeping, Dreaming, and Dying*, Wisdom Publications, 1997, p.45

5. Rob Nairn, *Living, Dreaming, Dying*, Shambhala Publications, 2004, p.194

6. *Ibid.*

7. B. Alan Wallace, *Dreaming Yourself Awake*, Shambhala, 2012, p.68

8. Varela and HH Dalai Lama, *op. cit.*, p.42

Chapter 5: The Spiritual Benefits of Lucid Dreaming

1.   Lama Yeshe Rinpoche in conversation with the author, June 2011

2.   Dzogchen Ponlop Rinpoche, *Mind Beyond Death*, Snow Lion Publications, 2008, p.1

3.   Michael Katz, *Tibetan Dream Yoga*, Bodhi Tree, 2011, p.37

4.   *Ibid.*, p.103

5.   B. Alan Wallace, *Dreaming Yourself Awake*, Shambhala Publications, 2012, p.20

6.   Chokyi Nyingma Rinpoche, Rigpa, London, 2010

7.   Dzigar Kongtrul Rinpoche, *It's Up to You*, Shambhala Publications, 2006, p.12

8.   Wallace, *op. cit.*, p.77

9.   Rob Nairn in conversation with the author, August 2011

10. Marcus Chown, 'Bonkers Things about the World', Science Museum, London; https://blog.sciencemuseum.org.uk/10-bonkers-things-about-the-world/ [accessed 15 March 2024]

11. Cited in Katz, *op. cit.*, p.120

12. Timothy Freke, teaching at Glastonbury Abbey, December 2010

13. Tenzin Wangyal Rinpoche, 'Dream Yoga', Ligmincha International, YouTube, 2010; http://www.youtube.com/watch?v=6Gls65GDMGQ [accessed 5 September 2023]

14. Steve Bradt, 'Wandering mind not a happy mind', *Harvard Gazette*, 11 November 2010; http://news.harvard.edu/gazette/story/2010/11/wandering-mind-not-a-happy-mind/ [accessed 5 September 2023]

15. Freke, *op. cit.*

Chapter 6: Daytime Lucid Dreaming Techniques

1.   Lama Surya Das, *Tibetan Dream Yoga*, audio CD, Sounds True, 2001

2.   Richard Wiseman, *59 Seconds*, Pan, 2010, p.16

3.   Unless there is damage to the multi-modal sensory cortex due to a stroke or head injury, as mentioned earlier, and even then, after recovery, dreams will return.

4.   Wiseman, *op. cit.*

5.   Carlos Castaneda, *Journey to Ixtlan*, Simon and Schuster, 1972, p.114

6.   *Ibid.*

7.   Kristen LaMarca, PhD, 'To lucid dream test your state by re-reading', 6 February 2018; https://www.mindfulluciddreaming.com/post/2018/02/05/rereading-state-test [accessed 12 April 2024]

8.   Jill Bolte Taylor, *My Stroke of Insight*, Hodder and Stoughton, 2008

9.   Wiseman, *op. cit.*

10. Matthew Walker, *The Tim Ferriss Show Transcripts:* 'Dr Matthew Walker, All Things Sleep Continued'; https://tim.blog/2023/02/10/dr-matthew-walker-transcript/ [accessed 16 April 2024]

11. Daniel Love, *Are You Dreaming?*, Enchanted Loom Publishing, 2013, p.2

12. *Ibid.*, p.83

13. Michael Katz, *Tibetan Dream Yoga*, Bodhi Tree, 2011, p.67, commenting on Gyaltrul Rinpoche, *Ancient Wisdom*, Snow Lion Publications, 1993, p.80

14. Akong Tulku Rinpoche in conversation with the author, 2009

15. Rob Nairn, teaching at Kagyu Samye Dzong Buddhist Centre, London, 2009

16. *Ibid.*

17. Bhante Henepola Gunaratana, 'Mindfulness and concentration', *Tricycle* online magazine, Fall 1998

18. Akong Tulku Rinpoche in conversation with the author, 2009

19. This research is currently unpublished, but was presented to participants of my online course 'Superlucid' in February 2022.

Chapter 7: Lucidity in Action: Top 10 Dream Plans

1.   Robert Waggoner, *Lucid Dreaming*, Moment Point Press, 2009, p.31

2.   Akong Tulku Rinpoche in conversation with the author, 2009

3.   Some lineages talk of three stages, others of six, but pretty much all of them contain the transmutation of fear, multiplication of phenomena and unification with the deity.

4.   Glenn H. Mullin, *Six Yogas of Naropa: Tsongkhapa's Commentary Entitled: A Book of Three Inspirations*, Snow Lion Publications, 2005

5.   Saljay Rinpoche, quoted in Yongey Mingyur, *Turning Confusion into Clarity: A Guide to the Foundation Practices of Tibetan Buddhism*, Snow Lion Publications, 2014, p.152

6.   Traleg Kyabgon Rinpoche, *Dream Yoga*, five-disc DVD set, E-Vam Buddhist Institute, 2008

7. Lama Yeshe Rinpoche in conversation with the author, July 2016

8. Ian Baker, in conversation with the author

9. Mullin, *op. cit.*

10. Namkhai Norbu Rinpoche, *The Cycle of Day and Night*, Barrytown/ Stationhill Press, 1987

11. Rob Nairn in conversation with the author, 2010

12. Akong Tulku Rinpoche in conversation with the author, 2009

13. B. Alan Wallace, teaching at the Kagyu Samye Dzong Buddhist Centre, London, June 2012

14. C.G. Jung, *The Archetypes and the Collective Unconscious* in *Collected Works* 9, Part I, Routledge and Kegan Paul, 1959

15. David Richo, *Shadow Dance: Liberating the Power and Creativity of Your Dark Side*, Shambhala Publications, 1999

16. Charlie Morley, TED talk, 2011

17. Kyabje Lama Zopa Rinpoche, *Abiding in the Retreat: A Nyung Na commentary*, ed. Ven. Ailsa Cameron; https://www.lamayeshe.com/ article/chapter/6-benefits-reciting-om-mani-padme-hum [accessed 25 April 2024]

Chapter 8: Night-time Lucid Dreaming Techniques

1. B. Alan Wallace, *Dreaming Yourself Awake*, Shambhala Publications, 2012, p.102

2. National Institutes of Health, 'How sleep clears the brain', *NIH Research Matters*, 28 October 2013; www.nih.gov/news-events/ nih-research-matters/how-sleep-clears-brain [accessed 12 April 2024]

3. Peters, B., 'How to resolve a lack of deep sleep'; www.verywellhealth.com/lack-of-deep-sleep-3966027 [accessed 12 April 2024]

4. Matthew Walker, *Joe Rogan Experience* #1109, 25 April 2018; www.youtube.com/watch?v=pwaWilO_Pig [accessed 12 April 2024]

5. Matthew Walker, *Why We Sleep*, Penguin, 2018, p.208

6. Quoted in Rob Nairn, *Living, Dreaming, Dying*, Shambhala Publications, 2004, p.38

7. *Ibid.*

8. Timothy Freke, 'Lucid Living' teachings, December 2009

9. Quoted in Francisco J. Varela and HH Dalai Lama, *Sleeping, Dreaming, and Dying*, Wisdom Publications, 1997, p.40

10. B. Alan Wallace, *Dreaming Yourself Awake*, Shambhala Publications, 2012, p.30

11. https://www.world-of-lucid-dreaming.com/mnemonic-induction-of-lucid-dreams.html [accessed 15 March 2024]

12. Erlacher, D., and Stumbrys, T., 'Wake up, work on dreams, back to bed and lucid dream: a sleep laboratory study', *Frontiers in Psychology* 11, 26 June 2020; https://pubmed.ncbi.nlm.nih.gov/32670163 [accessed 12 April 2024]

13. Cited by Traleg Kyabgon Rinpoche, *Dream Yoga*, five-disc DVD set, E-Vam Buddhist Institute, 2008

14. Wallace, *op. cit.*, p.99

15. Namgyal Rinpoche, *The Womb of Form*, Bodhi Publishing, 1998, p.73

16. Thubten Chodron; https://www.goodreads.com/quotes/817080-when-you-plant-seeds-in-the-garden-you-don-t-dig [accessed 12 April 2024]

Chapter 9: Liminal State Techniques

1. Carlos Castaneda, *Journey to Ixtlan*, Simon and Schuster, 1972

2. Mingyur Rinpoche, public talk, London, 2005

3. Hölzel, B.K., *et al.*, 'Mindfulness practice leads to increases in regional brain gray matter density', *Psychiatry Research* 191(1), 30 January 2011, 36–43; https://www.ncbi.nlm.nih.gov/pmc/articles/PMC3004979/ [accessed 12 April 2024]

4. Jeff Warren, *The Head Trip*, Oneworld Publications, 2009, p.39

5. Richard Wiseman, *59 Seconds*, Pan, 2010, p.119

6. Cited in Deirdre Barrett, *The Committee of Sleep*, Crown, 2001

7. Rob Nairn in conversation with the author, 2012

8. Krishnamurti, *The Beginnings of Learning*, Krishnamurti Foundation Trust, 1979

9. S. Hegarty, 'The myth of the eight-hour sleep', 22 February 2012; www.bbc.co.uk/news/magazine-16964783 [accessed 30 June 2021]

10. Clark Strand, 'Green meditation: the recovery of the dark', *Tricycle* online magazine, March 2010; www.tricycle.com/online-retreats/green-meditation/recovery-dark [accessed 5 September 2023]

11. Quoted in Liesa Goins, 'How to sleep right, tonight', *Men's Health*, 19 July 2012; https://www.menshealth.com/health/a19521803/sleep-right-tonight/ [accessed 5 September 2023]

12. Catherine Milner, *et al.*, 'Habitual napping moderates motor performance improvements following a short daytime nap', *Biological Psychology* 73(2), August 2006, 141–56; www.ncbi.nlm.nih.gov/pubmed/16540232 [accessed 5 September 2023]

13. 'Regular midday snoozes tied to a healthier heart', *The New York Times*, 13 February 2007; https://www.nytimes.com/2007/02/13/health/13nap.html [accessed 12 April 2024]

14. Karl Doghramji, MD, 'Melatonin and its receptors: a new class of sleep-promoting agents', *Journal of Clinical Sleep Medicine* 3(5 Suppl), 15 August 2007; https://jcsm.aasm.org/doi/full/10.5664/jcsm.26932 [accessed 15 March 2024]

15. Carlos Castaneda, *Journey to Ixtlan*, Simon and Schuster, 1972, p.127

Chapter 10: Embracing the Obstacles of the Night

1. Samuel Johnson; https://www.brainyquote.com/quotes/samuel_johnson_385293 [accessed 5 September 2023]

2. Lama Zangmo in conversation with the author, May 2011

3. John Greenleaf Whittier, 'Maud Muller', 1856

4. European Science Foundation, 'New links between lucid dreaming and psychosis could revive dream therapy in psychiatry', *Science Daily*, 29 July 2009; https://www.sciencedaily.com/releases/2009/07/090728184831.htm [accessed 5 September 2023]

5. Mota-Rolim, S.A., and Araujo, J.F., 'Neurobiology and clinical implications of lucid dreaming', *Medical Hypotheses* 81(5), November 2013, 751–6; www.ncbi.nlm.nih.gov/pubmed/23838126 [accessed 5 September 2023]

6. Cited in Matthew Walker, *Why We Sleep*, Penguin, 2018, p.211

7. Cited in Antti Revonsuo, 'Why Do We Dream?', *Horizon*, BBC TV, 21 February 2009

8. *Ibid.*

9. *Ibid.*

10. J. Allan Hobson, *Dreaming*, Oxford University Press, 2005

11. Paul and Charla Devereux, *Lucid Dreaming*, Daily Grail Publishing, 2011, p.177

Chapter 11: Treating PTSD Lucidly

1. This wonderful phrase is taken from the teachings of Robert Moss.

2. Els van der Helm, 'Dreaming takes the sting out of painful memories, research shows', *Science Daily*, 27 November 2011; https://www.sciencedaily.com/releases/2011/11/111123133346.htm [accessed 12 April 2024]

3. Yount, G., *et al.*, (2023). 'Decreased posttraumatic stress disorder symptoms following a lucid dream healing workshop', *Traumatology*, advance online publication; https://doi.org/10.1037/trm0000456 [accessed 22 March 2024]

Chapter 12: Blurring the Boundaries

1. Glenn H. Mullin, *Six Yogas of Naropa: Tsongkhapa's Commentary Entitled: A Book of Three Inspirations*, Snow Lion Publications, 2005

2. Michael Katz, *Tibetan Dream Yoga*, Bodhi Tree, 2011, p.8

3. *Ibid.*, p.40

4. C.G. Jung (ed.), *Man and his Symbols*, Aldus Books, 1964, p.37

5. Robert McLuhan, 'Precognitive dreaming should not be dismissed as coincidence', *Guardian*, 1 March 2011; https://www.theguardian.com/commentisfree/2011/mar/01/precognitive-dreaming-dismissed-science [accessed 5 September 2023]

6. Sturges, F., 'The Premonitions Bureau by Sam Knight review – astonishing adventures in precognition', 4 May 2022; https://www.theguardian.com/books/2022/may/04/the-premonitions-bureau-by-sam-knight-review-astonishing-adventures-in-precognition [accessed 12 April 2024]

7. Stowell, M.S., 'Precognitive dreams: a phenomenological study. Part I: Methodology and sample cases', *Journal of the American Society for Psychical Research* 91, 1997, 163–220

8. Cited by Dr Larry Dossey, Scientific and Medical Network conference, Winchester University, April 2011

9. 'Precognitive Stock Market Dreamers', *Phenomena*, 1 November 2004

10. Dossey, *op. cit.*

11. *Ibid.*

12. *Ibid.*

13. Quoted in 'Is this REALLY proof that man can see into the future?', *Daily Mail*, 4 May 2007; http://www.dailymail.co.uk/sciencetech/

article-452833/Is-REALLY-proof-man-future.html [accessed 5 September 2023]

14. NASA: 'Dark Energy, Dark Matter'; http://science.nasa.gov/astrophysics/focus-areas/what-is-dark-energy/ [accessed 5 September 2023]

15. Larry Dossey, MD, *The Power of Premonitions*, Hay House, 2009

16. Michael Katz, *Tibetan Dream Yoga*, Bodhi Tree, 2011, p.37

17. Dossey, *op. cit.*

18. *Ibid.*

19. Guterstam, A., *et al.*, 'The illusion of owning a third arm', *PLoS ONE* 6(2): e17208, online February 2011

20. Olivé, I., and Berthoz, A., 'Combined induction of rubber-hand illusion and out-of-body experiences', *Frontiers in Psychology* 3, 31 May 2012

21. B. Alan Wallace, UK Retreat, Lampeter, Wales, 2019

22. Published in his book *Flight of Mind*, Scarecrow Press, 1985

23. Thomas Campbell, *My Big TOE*, Lightning Strike Books, 2007, p.85

24. LaBerge, S., *Lucid Dreaming: The Power of Being Awake and Aware in Your Dreams*, Tarcher, 1985

25. Akong Rinpoche in conversation with the author, 2010

26. Francisco J. Varela and HH Dalai Lama, *Sleeping, Dreaming, and Dying*, Wisdom Publications, 1997

27. Andrew Holecek, *Dream Yoga*, Sounds True, 2016

Chapter 13: Beyond Lucidity

1. Timothy Freke teaching on gnosis, December 2011

2. Fritjof Capra, *The Tao of Physics*; http://www.goodreads.com/quotes/75791-quantum-theory-thus-reveals-a-basic-oneness-of-the-universe [accessed 5 September 2023]

3. Christopher Potter, *You Are Here*, Windmill Press, 2010, p.51

4. Werner Heisenberg, *Physics and Philosophy*, Harper and Row, 1962, p.145

5. Quoted in Werner Heisenberg, *Physics and Beyond: Encounters and Conversations*, Allen and Unwin, 1971, p.206

6. Adyashanti teachings

7. Rob Nairn, *Tranquil Mind*, Kairon Press, 1994

8. Pema Chödrön, 'No Right, No Wron', *Tricycle* online magazine, 1993; https://tricycle.org/magazine/no-right-no-wrong/ [accessed 12 April 2024]
9. Nairn, *op. cit.*
10. Dr Beau Lotto, 'Is Seeing Believing?', *Horizon*, BBC2, 8 January 2011
11. Dr Gustav Kuhn, *ibid.*
12. Dr Beau Lotto, *ibid.*
13. Traleg Kyabgon Rinpoche, *Dream Yoga*, five-disc DVD set, E-Vam Buddhist Institute, 2008
14. Lama Yeshe Rinpoche in conversation with the author, September 2012
15. BBC News, 'People spend "half their waking hours daydreaming"', 12 November 2010; www.bbc.co.uk/news/health-11741350 [accessed 5 September 2023]
16. Schuman-Olivier, Z., et al., 'Mindfulness and behavior change', *Harvard Review of Psychiatry* 28(6), Nov–Dec 2020, 371–94; https://www.ncbi.nlm.nih.gov/pmc/articles/PMC7647439/ [accessed 12 April 2024]
17. Stephen Batchelor, *Buddhism without Beliefs*, Riverhead Books, 1997, p.32
18. Dilgo Khyentse Rinpoche, 'A city of dreams', *Tricycle* online magazine, Spring 2007; https://tricycle.org/magazine/city-dreams [accessed 12 April 2024]
19. Tenzin Wangyal Rinpoche, London talk, November 2012

Chapter 14: Awakening within the Dream

1. Dilgo Khyentse Rinpoche, 'A city of dreams', *Tricycle* online magazine, Spring 2007; https://tricycle.org/magazine/city-dreams [accessed 12 April 2024]

Appendix I: Mindfulness Meditation

1. Cited in Richard Wiseman, *59 Seconds*, Pan, 2010
2. Tenzin Wangyal Rinpoche, 'Dream Yoga', Ligmincha International, YouTube, 2010: http://www.youtube.com/watch?v=6Gls65GDMGQ [accessed 5 September 2023]
3. Dzogchen Ponlop Rinpoche, *Mind Beyond Death*, Snow Lion Publications, 2008

BIBLIOGRAPHY

Valerie Austin, *Self-Hypnosis: A step-by-step guide to improving your life*, Thorsons, 1994

Marc Barasch, *Healing Dreams*, Riverhead, 2000

Deirdre Barrett, *The Committee of Sleep*, Crown, 2001

Stephen Batchelor, *Buddhism without Beliefs: A contemporary guide to awakening*, Riverhead Books, 1997

—, 'Buddhism for this one and only life', the first talk of his *Tricycle* online retreat, 26 June 2010

Fraser Boa, *The Way of the Dream: Conversations on Jungian dream interpretation with Marie-Louise von Franz*, Windrose, 1988

Joseph Campbell, *The Inner Reaches of Outer Space*, A. van der Marck, 1986

Thomas Campbell, *My Big TOE: Awakenings, discovery, inner workings: a trilogy unifying philosophy, physics, and metaphysics*, Lightning Strike Books, 2007

Fritjof Capra, *The Tao of Physics: An exploration of the parallels between modern physics and Eastern mysticism*, Shambhala Publications, 1975

Carlos Castaneda, *Journey to Ixtlan: The lessons of Don Juan*, Simon and Schuster, 1972

—, *The Art of Dreaming*, HarperCollins, 1994

Lama Surya Das, *Tibetan Dream Yoga*, audio CD, Sounds True, 2001

Paul and Charla Devereux, *Lucid Dreaming: Accessing your inner virtual realities*, Daily Grail Publishing, 2011

Larry Dossey, MD, *The Power of Premonitions*, Hay House, 2009

Debbie Ford, *The Shadow Effect: A Journey from Your Darkest Thought to Your Greatest Dream*, DVD, Hay House, 2009

Timothy Freke and Peter Gandy, *The Laughing Jesus*, Three Rivers Press, 2006

Sigmund Freud, *The Interpretation of Dreams*, trans. A.A. Brill, Macmillan, 1913; first published Franz Deuticke, 1899

Keith Hearne, *The Dream Machine*, Aquarian Press, 1990

Werner Heisenberg, *Physics and Philosophy*, Harper and Row, 1962

—, *Physics and Beyond: Encounters and conversations*, Allen and Unwin, 1971

J. Allan Hobson, *Dreaming: A very short introduction*, Oxford University Press, 2005

Andrew Holecek, *Dream Yoga*, Sounds True, 2016

Jim Horne, *Sleepfaring: A journey through the science of sleep*, Oxford University Press, 2006

H.J. Irwin, *Flight of Mind: A psychological study of the out-of-body experience*, Scarecrow Press, 1985

C.G. Jung, 'The importance of the unconscious in psychopathology', *British Medical Journal*, 2(2,814), 5 December 1914, 964–8

—, *Psychology and Religion*, 1938, in *Psychology and Religion: West and East; Collected Works*, Vol. 11, Princeton University Press, 1975

—, *Archetypes and the Collective Unconscious; Collected Works*, Vol. 9, Part 1, Routledge and Kegan Paul, 1959

— (ed.), *Man and his Symbols*, Aldus Books, 1964

—, *Dreams*, trans. R.F.C. Hull, Princeton University Press, 1974

Michael Katz, *Tibetan Dream Yoga: The royal road to enlightenment*, Bodhi Tree, 2011

Stephen LaBerge, PhD, *Lucid Dreaming*, Jeremy P. Tarcher, Inc., 1985

—, *Lucid Dreaming: A concise guide to awakening in your dreams and in your life*, Sounds True, 2004

— and Howard Rheingold, *Exploring the World of Lucid Dreaming*, Ballantine Books, 1990

Daniel Love, *Are You Dreaming? Exploring lucid dreams: a comprehensive guide*, Enchanted Loom Publishing, 2013

Robert A. Monroe, *Journeys Out of the Body*, Doubleday, 1971

Glenn H. Mullin, *Six Yogas of Naropa: Tsongkhapa's commentary entitled: A Book of Three Inspirations*, Snow Lion Publications, 2005

Rubin Naiman, PhD, *The Yoga of Sleep: Sacred and scientific practices to heal sleeplessness*, Sounds True, 2010

Rob Nairn, *Tranquil Mind: An introduction to Buddhism and meditation*, Kairon Press, 1994

—, *Living, Dreaming, Dying: Practical wisdom from the Tibetan Book of the Dead*, Shambhala Publications, 2004

David N. Neubauer, *Understanding Sleeplessness*, Johns Hopkins University Press, 2003

Chogyal Namkhai Norbu, *The Cycle of Day and Night: An essential Tibetan text on the practice of Dzogchen*, Barrytown/Stationhill Press, 1987

—, *Dream Yoga and the Practice of Natural Light*, Snow Lion Publications, 2002

Christopher Potter, *You Are Here: A portable history of the universe*, Windmill Press, 2010

Rob Preece, *The Psychology of Buddhist Tantra*, Snow Lion Publications, 2012

David Richo, *Shadow Dance: Liberating the power and creativity of your dark side*, Shambhala Publications, 1999

Dzigar Kongtrul Rinpoche, *It's Up to You*, Shambhala Publications, 2006

Dzogchen Ponlop Rinpoche, *Mind Beyond Death*, Snow Lion Publications, 2008

Gyaltrul Rinpoche, *Ancient Wisdom: Nyingma teachings of dream yoga, meditation and transformation*, Snow Lion Publications, 1993

Namgyal Rinpoche, *The Womb of Form: Pith instructions in the Six Yogas of Naropa*, Bodhi Publishing, 1998

Patrul Rinpoche, *Words of My Perfect Teacher: A complete translation of a classic introduction to Tibetan Buddhism*, trans. Padmakara Translation Group, Shambhala Publications, 1994

Tenzin Wangyal Rinpoche, *The Tibetan Yogas of Dream and Sleep*, Snow Lion Publications, 1998

Traleg Kyabgon Rinpoche, *Dream Yoga*, five-disc DVD set, E-Vam Buddhist Institute, 2008

G. Scott Sparrow, *Lucid Dreaming: Dawning of the clear light*, ARE Press, 1976

Jill Bolte Taylor, *My Stroke of Insight: A brain scientist's personal journey*, Hodder and Stoughton, 2008

Frederick van Eeden, 'A study of dreams', *Proceedings of the Society for Psychical Research*, 1913

Francisco J. Varela and HH Dalai Lama, *Sleeping, Dreaming, and Dying: An exploration of consciousness with the Dalai Lama*, Wisdom Publications, 1997

Robert Waggoner, *Lucid Dreaming: Gateway to the inner self*, Moment Point Press, 2009

B. Alan Wallace, *Dreaming Yourself Awake: Lucid dreaming and Tibetan dream yoga for insight and transformation*, Shambhala Publications, 2012

Jeff Warren, *Head Trip: A fantastic romp through 24 hours in the life of your brain*, Oneworld Publications, 2009

Richard Wiseman, *59 Seconds: Think a little, change a lot*, Pan, 2010

W.B. Yeats, *Responsibilities*, Cuala Press, 1914

Serenity Young, *Dreaming in the Lotus: Buddhist narrative, imagery and practice*, Wisdom Publications, 1999

ACKNOWLEDGEMENTS

The acknowledgements section from the 2013 edition of this book was pages long and the process of thanking people from the 10 years between then and now feels overwhelming and impossible. There are simply too many to thank.

My mission is to spread the dharma of the dream state into the West, just as Guru Padmasambhava did in Tibet, so if you have ever attended one of my courses or read one of my books, then I thank you for helping with this mission…

I would also like to express my gratitude to all the people who have helped me write this book and helped me be everything I can be. I take full responsibility for any errors or inaccuracies within the text and I apologize for any and all of these.

Huge thanks to my mum, dad, brother, Chloë, Waffles, Bao and stepfamily who have been so supportive over the past few years.

To Lama Zangmo and to all the London Samye Dzong sangha and to all the Samye Dzong centres at which I have had the privilege to teach.

To my dreams and to the hypnopompic state in which I composed many of the key points of this book.

To my teachers Lama Yeshe Rinpoche, Akong Rinpoche, Rob Nairn and Lama Zangmo for their kindness and patience with me.

To Rigpa and Sogyal Rinpoche for those first vital steps along the path. Thank you to my friends: Mantis Clan, Robbie C, Zia, Dynamic Stag, Donna, Jade, Millie and the Chaotic Pond Otters.

Thank you to Leah for her PR, Vishen and Mindvalley for the amazing new adventures and Awake Academy for the courses.

To Michelle, Jo, Julie, Lizzie and the rest of the brilliant team at Hay House for all their hard work.

And finally, thank *you* for taking the time to read this book. I sincerely hope that it benefits you in some way and that it encourages you to follow your dreams, as it did for me through writing it.

INDEX

A

acceptance 40–41, 119, 239–41
addictions 38
affirmations 134–9
    bodhicitta affirmation 135–6
    dream plan affirmation 138
    Toltec affirmation 137–8
Akong Rinpoche 95, 96, 111–12, 220, 221
alcohol 36–7
alien abductions, sleep paralysis and 189n
alpha waves 128
analytic psychology and shadow integration
    40–42
anxiety
    performance anxiety 180–83
    PTSD (post-traumatic stress disorder)
        193–203
archetypes
    interaction with internal 8, 197
    psycho-spiritual 49
    wisdom 61–2
astral projection see out-of-body
        experiences (OBEs)
Austin, Valerie 30
awakening see spiritual awakening; waking
        from sleep
awareness 4–6, 9, 15
    dream awareness 10–12, 13n, 31, 95–6
    see also Mindfulness of Dream &
        Sleep

in dreamless sleep 133
and 'flow-state' activities 19
and lucid living 233–41
mindfulness meditation see mindfulness
    meditation
Ayang Rinpoche 164n

B

balance 19, 154
Barasch, Marc 31
bardo states 50–51, 56, 107–8, 125
Barker, John 207
Barnard, E.E. xiii
Batchelor, Stephen 45, 238
Berkeley, George, Bishop 227n
Bernard, Arthur 208
bodhicitta 69
    bodhicitta affirmation 135–6
bodily illusions 213
bodily spasms 128
Body and Breath technique 147–8
Bohr, Niels 228, 232
Bön 48
brain
    chemical changes during phases of
        sleep 200
    cortex activation 4, 5–6, 26, 201
    hemispheres 17–18, 88, 162
    imaging technology 5

brain (continued)
increased brain frequency in lucid
dreams 9
neural pathways 6, 26, 27, 42, 58, 85–8,
113, 114
neuroplasticity 6, 26
physiology in lucid dreaming 4–6, 9,
24–5, 26, 42, 85–8, 114
and reality checking 85, 86–8
size 26
and sleep paralysis 188–90
and trauma integration 199–201
see also neuroscience
brainwaves
alpha 128, 170, 215
delta 129, 131, 133, 140, 171
gamma 9
theta 128, 129
breathing: Body and Breath technique
147–8
Buddha 7, 18, 45, 47, 48, 53, 100, 175,
244–5
Buddha nature 61, 105, 268–9
Buddha Nature Lucid! 268–9
Buddhism 139–42
and ignorance 49
and illusion 49, 233
karma 230–31
mantras 273–6, 277–8
role of dreams in 48–53
schools 47
and shunyata (emptiness) 60–61
see also emptiness (shunyata)
Tantric 49n, 124–5
teachings on how to wake up
46–7
Tibetan/Vajrayana see Tibetan
Buddhism/Vajrayana

C
Campbell, Thomas 216
careers: Career Path Lucidity 270–72
Castaneda, Carlos 86n, 92, 171
Celtic tradition 62
cerebrospinal fluid 129
chakras 277

Chenrezig 58
Chenrezig dream yoga 123–6
Lucid Self-Manifestation as Chenrezig
259–60
Chenrezig dream yoga: walking meditation
253–5
chi gong 58, 210
childhood trauma 33
see also inner child healing
Chödron, Pema 231
clarity dreams 52
Amazing Clarity Dream 257–8
Lama Yeshe Clarity Dream 269
Lucid Clarity Dream: The Final Teaching
from Rob 285–6
clear light experiences 52, 133
Guru Rinpoche Clear Light Lucid Dream
283–4
clear light of sleep 98
Cleveland Clinic Foundation 25
coincidences 237
collective unconscious 30n
Columbo method 93–4
compassion 47, 62, 69, 123–4, 227
see also Chenrezig
confabulation 92–3
confidence 182
conscious sleep
and astral projection see out-of-body
experiences (OBEs)
and the bardo states 50–51, 56,
220
clear light of sleep see falling asleep
consciously (FAC)
lucidity in dreaming see lucid dreaming
practice; lucid dreaming techniques;
lucid dreams
mindfulness in falling-asleep state see
hypnagogic mindfulness
mindfulness in waking-up period see
hypnopompic mindfulness
OBEs see out-of-body experiences
(OBEs)
techniques for mindfulness in sleep see
Mindfulness of Dream & Sleep
in Tibetan Buddhism and dream yoga
48–9, 51–3, 56, 57, 149

consciousness
blurring of boundary between personal and universal 205–6
Buddhism and the states of 51
see also *bardo* states
co-creating reality 229–30
delusion of 10
experiences of pure consciousness 164
lucid 4–6, 12, 205–6, 227
see also lucid dreams
lucid living 233–41
out-of-body see out-of-body experiences (OBEs)
and physical 'reality' 7–10, 228–40
reflective 6, 10
the shared dream 232
union of 49
Constantine 206
control 13–15
counting sleep 148
creativity
co-creating reality 229–30
hypnagogic 162–3
and integrating the shadow 118
and lucid dreaming 17–18

D
Dalai Lama 50, 53, 144, 199, 220
Dali, Salvador 163
dancing 253, 254n
and lucid dreams 19
dead, communicating with 106–9
death
contemplation of 238
in lucid dream examples 281
preparation for 50–51, 55–7, 109–10
deep sleep 129–30
deity self-visualization 58, 124–6
Guru Rinpoche Self-manifestation and Lama Yeshe, OBE! 277–8
Lucid Self-Manifestation as Chenrezig 259–60
delta waves 129
Dement, William 188
depression, curing 34–5

Devereux, Paul 214
diary keeping 71–2
Dossey, Larry 208–9
dozing see hypnagogic mindfulness
dream body 57–8, 154, 220, 221, 260
dream characters 12, 14, 92, 104n
in lucid dream examples 258, 259, 261, 262, 263–4, 266–7, 270–71, 272–3, 273–5, 276–7, 277–8, 279–80, 280–81, 284–5, 285–6
and nightmares 187
and shadow integration 119, 120
dream diaries 71–2
benefits of 80–81
dating 80n
top tips 81–2
Dream Initiated Lucid Dream (DILD) 85
dream plan affirmation 138
dream planning 70, 73–7, 172
creating a *sankalpa* (intention setting) 74–5
drawing 74
threefold manifestation 76–7
top 10 plans 99–126
and trauma resolution 197–8
writing 74
dream recall 71, 77–80, 172
boosting 78–80
and diary keeping 71–2
dream signs 72, 83–5, 172–3
spotting 83–5
dream telepathy 206–12
see also prophetic dreams
dream yoga 48–50, 56, 57, 67–8, 110, 149
Chenrezig dream yoga 123–6
Lucid Self-Manifestation as Chenrezig 259–60
stages of 109, 110
dreams/dreaming
and alcohol 36–7
clarity dreams 52, 257–8, 265–6, 269, 285–6
and clear light experiences 133
and communication with the unconscious 15–16, 37–8
control of 13–15

dreams/dreaming (continued)
  dream awareness 10–12, 13n, 31, 95–6
    see also Mindfulness of Dream &
      Sleep
  dreaming reality into existence 229–30
  examples 257–86
  and ignorance 49
  lucid see lucid dreams
  mindfulness of dream and sleep see
    Mindfulness of Dream & Sleep
  and neuroscience see neuroscience
  and nicotine 38
  nightmares 38–40, 183–7
  projection in 8, 49, 64, 86, 87, 107, 108,
    153–4, 219, 258, 261, 272–3
  prophetic 206–12
  and psychoanalysis/analytic psychology
    40–42, 118, 119
  quantum dreaming 227–9
  reality of 7–10, 27
  recall see dream recall
  REM (rapid eye movement) sleep
    130–31
  samsaric 51–2
  the shared dream 232, 233–4
  signs that we are dreaming 72
  in Tibetan Buddhist practice 48–53
  transpersonal content 30n, 52
  witnessing 13
Drupon Rinpoche 221
Dzigar Kongtrul Rinpoche 60
Dzogchen Ponlop Rinpoche 55

E
Edison, Thomas 162–3
Eeden, Frederik van 4, 5
EEG (electroencephalography) 5, 21, 22,
  24–5, 170
Einstein, Albert 10, 232
Emerson, Ralph Waldo 99, 182
emptiness (shunyata) 60–61, 233
  of atoms 61, 227–8
  of the dream state 110–12
  and Oneness 227–8
  and projection 110–11, 226–31, 233
  and the shared dream of life 232, 233

energy work 58, 210
enlightenment see spiritual awakening
enthusiasm 182
European Science Foundation 184

F
falling asleep consciously (FAC) 144–8
  see also hypnagogic mindfulness
false awakenings 113, 191–2
  and OBEs 215
fear 109–10
  night terrors 188
  nightmares 183–7
  see also performance anxiety
flow-states 96–7
  and increased awareness 19
flying dreams 12, 14
Fox, Dr 243
Freke, Timothy 63, 272–3
Freud, Sigmund 30n, 205, 206
friendliness 46, 239–41
fun 42–3

G
Gackenbach, Jayne 19, 113
galaxies xiii
Gnosticism 63, 133, 226
Goldacre, Ben 37
Green, Celia 11
grief, letting go of 106–9, 116–17,
  284–5
Guru Padmasambhava 109, 134, 171
Guru Rinpoche 277–8
  Guru Rinpoche Clear Light Lucid Dream
    283–4

H
hallucinations 189
happiness 253n
Harary, Keith 216
healing 31–3, 113–15, 266, 284–5
  curing depression 34–5
  healing the body 35–8, 279–80
  healing the inner child 32–3, 74

trauma resolution 38–40, 184–7,
  193–203
Hearne, Keith 21–3
Hegel, Georg Wilhelm Friedrich 21
Heisenberg, Werner 228
Helm, Els van der 200
HGH (human growth hormone) 129–30
higher self see Buddha nature
Holecek, Andrew 220
hour of the wolf 167–9
Humphreys, Matt 34–5
hyperacusis 189
hyperventilation 189
hypnagogic imagery 128, 145–6, 147, 157,
  162–3, 218
hypnagogic mindfulness 159–62
  and creativity 162–3
  hypnagogic affirmation 134–9
  hypnagogic drop-in exercise 145–6
  and MILD (Mnemonic Initiated Lucid
    Dream) technique 139–42
  see also conscious sleep
hypnagogic state 71, 79, 128, 157–8
  and creativity 162–3
  hallucinations in 189
  and sleep paralysis 188–90
hypnopompic mindfulness 158, 164–6,
  169
hypnopompic state 131, 158
  insights in 158
  and sleep paralysis 188–90
hypnosis 30, 245–6
  self-hypnosis 71, 79

I
ignorance 49
illusion 49, 213, 233
Illusory Body yoga 237
imaginary rehearsal 100–102
impossibilities 243–4
Inception 43
individuation 41
inner child healing 32–3, 74, 115–17, 198,
  280
  Grief Healed Through the Inner Child
    284–5

insight 4, 45, 69, 164
  in dream yoga 49
  hypnopompic insights 158
insomnia 169n
  and the hour of the wolf 167–9
intentions, setting 68, 71, 74–5, 78, 79, 84, 141
  stating out loud 75n
  see also affirmations
interconnectivity 62, 209, 226–9, 231
intuition 17, 237
IONS study 195–203
Irwin, Harvey 215–16

J
Jesus Christ 61, 206
Josephson, Brian 209
Juan (Matus), Don 86n, 92
Jung, Carl Gustav 30n, 32, 40, 52, 118, 199,
  206–7

K
karma 43, 230–31
Katz, Michael 57
Kekulé, Friedrich 3
Khyentse, Dilgo, Rinpoche 238, 246
  Amazing Clarity Dream 257–8
kindness 46, 235, 239, 240
  *Lucid Clarity Dream: The Final Teaching
    from Rob* 285–6
knowledge
  unconscious library of 30–31
  "What is the Essence of All Knowledge?"
    265–6
Kolk, Bessel van der 201
Kozhevnikov, Maria 97
Krishnamurti, Jiddu 166

L
LaBerge, Stephen 22–4, 69
  Exploring the World of Lucid Dreaming
    140
  Lucidity Institute 85, 87
  Mnemonic Initiated Lucid Dream
    technique 139–42

Lawrence, T.E. 229
Levine, Peter A. 193
life rehearsal 100–102
life signs 237
light sleep 129
liminal state techniques
creating a practice 171–5
the hour of the wolf 167–9
hypnagogic creativity 162–3
hypnagogic mindfulness 159–62
hypnagogic state 157–8
hypnopompic mindfulness 164–6
napping 169–71
Lotto, Beau 232
Love, Daniel 90
lucid dreaming practice
activities 99–126
and alcohol 36–7
and asking 'big questions' 102–4
balancing detachment and participation 153–4
and being kind 239–41
benefits of 10, 15–16, 29–43, 55–64
and the brain see neuroscience
co-creating the dream 15, 231, 233
communication during 27
and confidence 182
and control of dreams 13–15
and creativity 17–18
cumulative training 180–81
curing depression 34–5
diary keeping 71–2
doing things that scare you 109–10
and dream yoga see dream yoga
embracing the obstacles 179–92
and emptiness 60–61
encouraging prophetic dreams 210–12
and enthusiasm 182
everyone's ability for 16–19
and the experience of Oneness 226–7
exploring the emptiness of the dream 110–12
and false awakenings 113, 191–2
as a form of mind training 4, 100–102
fun with 42–3
and gender 18
healing the body 35–8

healing the inner child 32–3
healing through 31–3, 113–15, 266, 279–80
inner child healing 115–17
interaction with internal archetypes 8, 197–8
learning during 28
letting go of grief 106–9
and life rehearsal 100–102
and lucid living 63–4, 68, 233–41
maintaining lucidity 151–6
and manifestation 229–30
and meditation 19, 58, 121–3, 258–9
see also Mindfulness of Dream & Sleep
and motivation 18, 42, 68–9
as a movement 245–7
and moving through dream boundaries 205–23
as natural 17
and neuroscience see neuroscience
and nightmares 38–40
and OBEs for spiritual growth 221–3
in preparation for death 50–51, 55–7
preparing the space 67–8
psychological benefits 29–43
and PTSD (post-traumatic stress disorder) 193–203
and receiving teachings 61–2, 261, 269
self-doubt in ability for 180–83
and shadow integration 40–42, 118–21, 262–3, 263–5, 274–5
and sleeping position 78
spiritual benefits 55–64
and spiritual practice 57–8, 221–3
see also spiritual awakening
and sports science 24–5
stating intent 75n
and surfing 146
techniques for see lucid dreaming techniques
as threat to egoic sense of self 92–3
and the throat chakra 277
time estimation in 24, 152n
and trauma integration 199–201
and trauma resolution 38–40, 184–7, 193–203

and the unconscious 15–16, 37–8
verification experiments 21–4, 26–7
visualization in 25, 36–8, 58
and walking through walls 110–13,
    276–7
lucid dreaming techniques 67–97
    arm rubbing and hand checking 154
    boosting lucidity 153
    Columbo method 93–4
    dream diaries 71–2
    dream planning 70, 73–7
    dream recall 71, 77–80
    dream signs 72, 83–5
    falling asleep consciously (FAC) 144–8
    flow states 96–7
    the four 'D's 70–85
    hypnagogic affirmation technique
        134–9
    'Keep Calm and Carry On!' technique
        152–3
    looking for weirdness 89–91
    for maintaining lucidity 151–6
    MILD (Mnemonic Initiated Lucid
        Dream) technique 139–42
    mindfulness meditation 95–6
    Mnemonic Initiated Lucid Dream
        technique 139–42
    multiple wake-ups technique 149–51
    pre-lucid confabulation 91–3
    reality checking 85–8, 93–4, 154
    recall boosting 71, 78–80
    and receiving teachings 105–6
    setting intentions 68, 71, 74–5, 75n,
        78, 79, 84
    spinning 154–6
    spotting dream signs 72, 83–5
    Tibetan dream yoga see dream yoga
    'Wake up back to bed' method 142–4
lucid dreams
    and brain physiology 4–6, 24–5, 42,
        85–8, 114
        see also neuroscience
    of Buddha nature 268–9
    Buddha Nature Lucid! 268–9
    of career path 270–72
    Career Path Lucidity 270–72
    of children 16–18

and dancing 19, 97
Ear-Infection Healing Dream 279–80
and the essence of all knowledge
    265–6
exploring the dreamscape 249–50,
    274–5
of flying 12, 14
as a form of mind training 5–6
Grief Healed Through the Inner Child
    284–5
Guru Rinpoche Clear Light Lucid Dream
    283–4
Guru Rinpoche Self-manifestation and
    Lama Yeshe, OBE! 277–8
of healing 113–15, 115–17, 266,
    279–80
'How Can I Be of Most Benefit?' 281–2
Huge Lucid Dream with Walking Through
    Walls and Entry into the Void 276–7
Huge 'Show Me Something Important'
    Lucid Dream! 280–81
and increased awareness 5–6, 15,
    233–41
Lama Yeshe Clarity Dream 269
letting go of grief 106–9
levels of lucidity see lucidity spectrum
Lucid Clarity Dream: The Final Teaching
    from Rob 285–6
Lucid Meditation 258–9
Lucid Self-Manifestation as Chenrezig
    259–60
meditation in 121–3, 258–9
Meeting my Subconscious Mind 266–8
meeting the subconscious mind 266–8
nature of 3–6
OBEs as unrecognised dreams 215
obstacles to 179–92
One Hundred-Syllable Mantra Lucid
    Dream 273–6
practice of see lucid dreaming practice
reading text in 87
receiving teachings 61–2, 105–6, 261,
    269
self-manifestation as Chenrezig 58,
    259–60
Shadow Integration 262–3
Shadow Integration Lucid Dream 263–5

lucid dreams (continued)
  shadow integration through 40–42,
    118–21, 262–3, 263–5, 274–5
  spontaneous 13n, 16
  Teachings from Lama Yeshe Rinpoche
    261–2
  Teachings on Pain and Suffering 272–3
  techniques see lucid dreaming
    techniques
  timing of 24
  using digital/electrical appliances in 87
  vs out-of-body experiences (OBEs)
    218–19
  and walking through walls 110–13
  "What is the Essence of All Knowledge?"
    265–6
lucid living 63–4, 68, 233–41
  and acceptance 239–40
  and friendliness 239–41
  and kindness 239–41
  and life signs 237
  and meditation 236
  and thinking about death 238
Lucidity Institute 85, 87
lucidity spectrum 10–16
  fully lucid state 12
  pre-lucid state 11
  semi-lucid state 11
  super-lucid state 12
  witnessing dreams 13
lucidity triggers 72, 84

M
Magaña, Sergio 137
magnetic resonance tomography (MRT) 5
manifestation
  *Guru Rinpoche Self-manifestation and
    Lama Yeshe, OBE!* 277–8
  Lucid Self-Manifestation as Chenrezig
    259–60
manifestation practices 229–30
mantras 124–6, 273–6, 277–8, 283–4
materialism, scientific 228–9
Matis, Don Juan 157
McKenzie, Keith 193, 194–5
McMoneagle, Joe 217

meditation 13n, 19, 47, 57–8, 121–3
  Body and Breath technique 147–8
  Chenrezig dream yoga 123–6
  on death 238
  in lucid dreams 121–3, 258–9
  and lucid living 236
  mindful see mindfulness meditation
  snooze button meditation see
    hypnopompic mindfulness
  walking 253–5
memory see dream recall
micro-awakenings 128, 132, 169, 217
MILD (Mnemonic Initiated Lucid Dream)
  technique 139–42
military veterans & personnel 193, 194–5
Mindfulness Association 96, 159, 249
mindfulness meditation 19, 47, 95–7,
    121–3
  Chenrezig dream yoga 123–6
  in falling-asleep state see hypnagogic
    mindfulness
  and reality checks 91
  sitting meditation 249–53
  training 61
  in waking-up period see hypnopompic
    mindfulness
  whilst walking 253–5
  see also Mindfulness of Dream & Sleep
Mindfulness of Dream & Sleep 67–97,
    127–75
  and balance improvement 19, 154
  basic techniques 67–97
  and being kind 46, 235, 239–41
  benefits of 10, 15–16, 29–43, 55–64
  Body and Breath technique 147–8
  clear light of sleep 133
  and confidence 182
  counting sleep 148
  and enthusiasm 182
  falling asleep consciously see falling
    asleep consciously (FAC)
  fun with 42–3
  hypnagogic affirmation 134–9
  hypnagogic drop-in exercise 145–6
  liminal state techniques 157–75
  lucid dreaming techniques see lucid
    dreaming techniques

mindfulness in falling-asleep state *see*
hypnagogic mindfulness
mindfulness in waking-up period *see*
hypnopompic mindfulness
multiple wake-ups technique 149–51
and napping 169–71
and prayer 122, 134
preparing the space 67–8
and sleep paralysis 155n, 190
and sleeping position 78
and the stages of sleep 128–31
step by step 172–5
Wake Initiated Lucid Dream (WILD)
technique 144
Mindrolling Rinpoche 220n
Mingyur Rinpoche 159
Mnemonic Initiated Lucid Dream (MILD)
technique 139–42
Monroe, Robert 226–7
Morpheus 225
motivation 18, 42, 68–9
MRT (magnetic resonance tomography) 5
multiple wake-ups technique 149–51
muscle-tone monitoring 25
myoclonic jerks 128

N
Nairn, Rob 29, 50–51, 61, 108, 111, 123n,
125, 164, 169n, 184, 249, 262, 263
*Lucid Clarity Dream: The Final Teaching
from Rob* 285–6
Namgyal Rinpoche 149
Namkai Norbu Rinpoche 37
napping 169–71
Naropa 49
Neubauer, David 168
neuroplasticity 6, 26
neuroscience 4–6, 21–4, 26–7
brain physiology during lucid dreaming
4–6, 24–5, 42, 85–8, 114, 140
and the purpose of dreaming 130–31
and reality checks 86–8
and trauma integration 199–201
neurotoxins 129
Nicholls, Graham 218
nicotine 38, 113

night terrors 188
nightmares 38–40, 117, 119, 183–7
and PTSD (post-traumatic stress
disorder) 193, 195–203
and trauma resolution 184–7
noradrenaline 200
Norbu, Namkai Rinpoche 62, 111
norepinephrine 200
NSDR (non-sleep deep rest) 159, 171

O
OBEs *see* out-of-body experiences (OBEs)
obstacles to lucid dreaming 180–83
Oneness 10, 226–31
see also interconnectivity
out-of-body experiences (OBEs) 212–23,
277–8
embodiment 219
entry 218–19
Locale 1 OBEs 214–15, 277–8
and lucid dreams for spiritual growth
221–3
malleability 220
and movement 218
scientific proof of 213–18
sleep-initiated 214–15, 214n
spotting an OBE 218–19
Tibetan Buddhist view 219–21
time estimation in 219
as unrecognised lucid dreams 215
vs lucid dreams 218–19

P
pain: *Teachings on Pain and Suffering* 272–3
Pali Vinaya 48
Patrul Rinpoche 133
Perceptual and Motor Skills 23
performance anxiety 180–83
phobias 37
placebo effect 36–7, 114
Poe, Edgar Allan 191, 205
Potter, Christopher 227n
prayer 122, 134
pre-lucid confabulation 91–3
precognitive dreams 208–12

Preece, Rob 15
premonition dreams 208–12
problem solving: hypnagogic state 162–3
projection
    astral see out-of-body experiences
        (OBEs)
    as a defence mechanism 64
    in dreams 8, 37, 64, 86, 87, 107,
        110–11, 130, 153–4, 219, 258,
        263–5, 272–3
    and emptiness of wakeful experience
        110–11, 226–31, 233
    of enlightened potential 62
    of the shadow see also shadow
        integration
    shared 233
prophetic dreams 206–12
    encouraging 210–12
prospective memory 140
'psychic spies' 217
psychoanalysis 31–3
psychophysiological arousal see flow-states
PTSD (post-traumatic stress disorder)
        193–203
    IONS study 195–203

Q
quantum dreaming 227–9
quantum physics 61, 227–9

R
rapid eye movement sleep see REM (rapid
        eye movement) sleep
reading: reality checks 87–8
reality
    co-creating 229–30
    dreaming reality into existence 229–30
reality checking 85–8, 93–4, 154, 172–3
    and false awakenings 192
    in waking state 89–91, 94
recall of dreams see dream recall
receiving teachings 61–2, 105–6, 261, 269
REM (rapid eye movement) sleep 5, 22,
        78, 130–31
    and alcohol 36–7

and hypnagogic mindfulness 163
and the MILD technique 140
during napping 170
and nicotine 38, 113
and night terrors 188
and nightmares 183
and OBEs 218
REM rebound 143
and sleep paralysis 188–90
and spinning 154–5
and trauma 199
and trauma integration 200, 201
retraumatization 199
Revonsuo, Antti 186
Richo, David 33, 118
Ruiz, Don Miguel 32–3

S
samsar and samsaric dreams 51–2
sankalpa see intentions, setting
School of Movement Medicine 254n
scientific materialism 228–9
scientific proof of OBEs 213–18
scientific research into lucid dreaming
        neurological see neuroscience
        verification experiments 21–4, 26–7
Scurry, James 196
self-deception 7
self-hypnosis 71, 79
self-visualization see deity self-visualization
shadow integration 40–42, 118–21, 262–3,
        263–5, 274–5
    Shadow Integration 262–3
    Shadow Integration Lucid Dream
        263–5
shunyata see emptiness (shunyata)
singing bowls 165n
sitting meditation 249–53
Six Yogas of Naropa 49
sleep
    and alcohol 36–7
    clear light of 52, 133
    conscious see conscious sleep;
        falling asleep consciously (FAC);
        hypnagogic mindfulness; Mindfulness
        of Dream & Sleep

counting 148
cycles 128–33
deep sleep 129–30
dreamless 133
and the hour of the wolf 167–9
hours per night 150, 173n
lack of 167–9
light sleep 129
mental images seen when falling asleep
   see hypnagogic imagery
napping 169–71
and nicotine 38, 113
non-aware 56, 63–4
paralysis 147, 163, 188–90
REM see REM (rapid eye movement)
   sleep
REM (rapid eye movement) sleep
   130–31
stages 128–31
   see also REM (rapid eye
      movement) sleep
two sleeps pattern 167
sleep paralysis 155n
sleep spindles 129
sleeping position 78
snoozing, hypnopompic mindfulness
   164–6
Sogyal Rinpoche 258
Sparrow, G. Scott 142
spinning 154–6
spiritual awakening 46–7, 235
   and the bardo states 50–51, 56
   embodiments of enlightenment
      61–2
      see also Buddha; Jesus Christ
   and the experience of Oneness
      226–7, 229
   Gnostic teachings 63, 133, 226
   lucid awakening within the shared
      dream of life 243–7
   lucid dreams and OBEs for spiritual
      growth 221–3
   prayer to enlightened beings 136
   receiving teachings from enlightened
      beings 61–2, 105–6, 261, 269
   of Siddhartha Gautama, to become the
      Buddha 45, 244–5

and spiritual practice 57–8, 221–3
   see also meditation; prayer
and wakefulness in Tibetan Buddhism
   52
sports science 24–5
stress 200
subconscious mind
   Meeting my Subconscious Mind 266–8
   meeting personification of 266–8
suffering: Teachings on Pain and Suffering
   272–3
synchronicities 237

T
tai chi 58, 97, 210
Tantra 15–16
Tao of Dozing see hypnagogic mindfulness
Taoist dream practitioners 170
Taylor, Alan 228n
Taylor, Cathryn L. 116
theta waves 128, 129
'thin places' (Celtic tradition) 62
throat chakra 277
Tibetan Book of the Dead 56
Tibetan Buddhism/Vajrayana 47, 48–53,
   57–8, 69
   bardos 50–51, 56, 107–9, 220
   bodhicitta affirmation 135–6
   Chenrezig dream yoga 123–6
   clear light experiences 52, 133
   dream yoga see dream yoga
   Illusory Body yoga 237
   and OBEs 219–21
   prophetic dreams 206
   role of dreams in 48–50, 51–3
   setting intentions 79
   Tibetan synthesis of Vajrayana and
      Bön 48
   wakefulness 52
time estimation
   in lucid dreaming 24
   in OBEs 219
Tolle, Eckhart 243
Toltec affirmation 137–8
transpersonal dream experiences 30n, 52
trauma resolution

and dream planning 197–8
inner child healing 32–3, 198
nightmares 38–40, 184–7
PTSD (post-traumatic stress disorder)
193–203
trauma integration 199–201
Tsongkhapa, Lama 62

U
unconditional friendliness 46, 239–40
unconscious, the 30–31
collective unconscious 30n
communication with 15–16, 26–8, 31,
37–8
and creativity 162–3
diving into 205–6
fear of interference with 15–16
and a library of knowledge 30–31
meeting the subconscious mind in a
lucid dream 266–8
and prophetic dreams 206–12
the shadow 45–7, 118–21, 262–3,
263–5, 274–5

V
Vajrayana see Tibetan Buddhism/Vajrayana
video gaming and flow state 96–7
visualization 25, 35–6, 52
deity self-visualization 58, 124–6
within lucid dreams 25, 36–8, 58, 141

W
Waggoner, Robert 9, 12, 14, 36, 100, 234
Wake Initiated Lucid Dream (WILD)
technique 144
'wake up, back to bed' method 142–4
waking from sleep
false awakenings 113, 215
micro-awakenings 128, 132, 217
mindfulness in waking-up period see
hypnopompic mindfulness
multiple wake-ups technique
149–51
spiritually see spiritual awakening

'wake up, back to bed' method
142–4
waking state
reality checking 89–91, 94
see also mindfulness meditation
and shadow integration 120n
Walker, Matthew xiii–xiv, 90, 131
walking meditation 253–5
walking through walls 110–13, 276–7
Wallace, B. Allan 51, 114, 127, 142, 215,
233
Wangyal Rinpoche, Tenzin 63, 252
Warren, Jeff 167, 168
weird technique 89–91, 173
Whitfield, Dr Charles 32
Whittier, John Greenleaf 183
WILD (Wake Initiated Lucid Dream)
technique 144
Wilde, Oscar 206
wisdom 47, 49
archetypes 61–2
and asking 'big questions' 102–4
and the essence of all knowledge
265–6
innate wisdom and receiving teachings
61–2, 105–6, 261, 269
see also insight
Wiseman, Richard 36–7, 82n, 249n
witnessing dreams 13
Worsley, Alan 21–2

Y
Yeats, W.B. 42
Yeshe Rinpoche 55, 56, 105, 109–10, 194,
219–20, 235, 259, 274
Guru Rinpoche Self-manifestation and
Lama Yeshe, OBE! 277–8
Lama Yeshe Clarity Dream 269
Teachings from Lama Yeshe Rinpoche
261–2
Yoga Nidra 159n
Yount, Dr Garret 195, 202

Z
Zangmo, Lama 182, 284–5

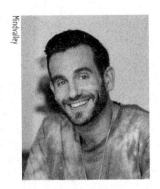

Mindvalley

ABOUT THE AUTHOR

Charlie Morley is a bestselling author and teacher of lucid dreaming, shadow integration and Mindfulness of Dream & Sleep.

He has been lucid dreaming for over 20 years and was 'authorized to teach' within the Kagyu school of Tibetan Buddhism by Lama Yeshe Rinpoche in 2008. Since then he has written four books, which have been translated into 15 languages, and has run workshops and retreats in more than 20 countries.

He has spoken at both Oxford and Cambridge Universities and run courses and given talks for the Metropolitan Police, Reuters News Agency and the Army Air Corps, as well as presenting his work with military veterans on Sky News and at the Ministry of Defence Mindfulness Symposium.

In 2018 he was awarded a Winston Churchill Fellowship to research PTSD treatment in military veterans and continues to teach workshops for people with trauma-affected sleep. These teachings form the core of his latest book, *Wake Up to Sleep*.

In 2019, in a world first, he trained a group of therapists to use lucid dreaming with their clients. An expanded and updated

100-hour version of this course ran again in 2023 under the title 'Lucid Dream Facilitator Training'.

In 2023, the first scientific study into Charlie's methods was published in the peer-reviewed journal *Traumatology*, in which 85 per cent of participants experienced 'a remarkable decrease in PTSD symptoms' through using lucid dreaming to transform their nightmares.

Charlie formally became a Buddhist at the age of 19, lived at the Kagyu Samye Dzong Buddhist centre for seven years and completed a three-month solitary meditation retreat at the Tara Rokpa centre in 2016.

He trained and worked as an actor and scriptwriter before running a hip-hop collective called THROWDOWN throughout his twenties.

He now lives in London with his partner, Chloë, and their two dogs, Waffles the wiener and Bao the Chow Chow. When he's not teaching, he enjoys kickboxing, surfing and pretending to meditate.

www.charliemorley.com

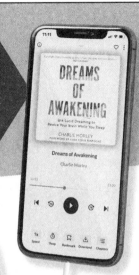

CONNECT WITH
HAY HOUSE
ONLINE

🌐 hayhouse.co.uk   **f** @hayhouse

📷 @hayhouseuk   𝕏 @hayhouseuk

▶ @hayhouseuk   ♪ @hayhouseuk

'*The gateways to wisdom and knowledge are always open.*'

Louise Hay